THE MIGRAINE GUIDE & COOKBOOK

The
Migraine Guide
&
Cookbook

JOSIE A. WENTWORTH

Introduction by
DR KATHARINA DALTON
MRCGP

SIDGWICK & JACKSON
LONDON

First published in Great Britain in 1981 by
Sidgwick and Jackson Limited

ISBN 0 283 98741 3

Typeset by Preface Ltd., Salisbury, Wilts.

Printed and bound in Great Britain by
Biddles Ltd., Guildford and King's Lynn
for Sidgwick and Jackson Limited
1 Tavistock Chambers, Bloomsbury Way
London WC1A 2SG

Acknowledgments

I WOULD like especially to thank Dr Katharina Dalton (whose idea this book originally was) for her constant support and help in supplying and checking material and her continued encouragement.

My thanks also go to my husband Peter for his constant help and making me stick at it; to my dear friend Megan Feachem who deciphered my handwriting and typed the manuscript; to my sister Jill F. Middleton for her general help with the recipe section and for the many recipes she supplied; and to John Holtom for endless hours checking and rechecking the typescript.

I am grateful also for the help given me by the following:

Cadbury Schweppes Limited (Research Laboratories)
Wendy M. Clark, Microbiologist, John Harvey & Sons, Wine Merchants, Bristol
The British Migraine Association
Dr Edda Hanington (Wellcome Trust)
British Medical Association
The Royal Society of Medicine
Journal of the Royal College of General Practitioners
Janet Maclean
Michael Bateman
Dr Saxby, British Food Manufacturers' Research Association

ACKNOWLEDGMENTS – *continued*

Jim Dawson
Office of Health Economics
Monica Shipp
Harcourt Brace & World Inc
George Allen & Unwin Ltd

Contents

CONTENTS

Introduction

MIGRAINE is a common and incapacitating disorder which is still listed among the diseases of unknown origin. Much research work is continuing throughout the world; every year more knowledge accumulates and little shafts of light are beginning to appear.

For a migraine attack to occur, certain conditions must first be satisfied. The individual must be susceptible to migraine (it is sometimes difficult to realise there are many lucky folk who have never experienced one). This susceptibility to migraines is usually already present at birth, being frequently inherited through one or other parent, or a grandparent. On the other hand, it may more rarely be acquired as a result of a severe head injury or meningitis. Then there are certain factors which make a susceptible individual more prone to develop attacks, and in this category come tension, stress, fatigue and lack of sleep. With women there are certain times when they are more liable to develop an attack; and these times include the few days before menstruation, the days during menstruation, immediately after childbirth, during the week off the contraceptive pill and at the menopause. Nevertheless, these factors only increase the tendency to develop a migraine. There still remain those final precipitating factors which trigger off a full-blown migraine attack. The best understood of the final trigger factors are the dietary ones. These include going for too long an interval between meals and eating specific foods of which the individual's enzyme system cannot dispose, so that certain substances – vaso-dilating amines – accumulate in the blood, and open wide the blood vessels of the brain, causing that intolerable throbbing headache.

While none of us can do anything about our parents or our family tree, and it is often hard to ensure freedom from tension, stress and lack of sleep, nevertheless it is possible to understand and eliminate the dietary factors which can trigger off an attack. Today there are many thousands of migraine patients who have successfully mastered the subject and have altered their eating habits so that they can now happily report long intervals between attacks. Indeed, some even speak of their rare attacks as having been 'self-induced', adding perhaps: 'I couldn't help it – the plane was delayed and no food was available' or 'It was such a lovely wedding, how could I say no to the champagne?'

This book fills a vital need in helping migraine-sufferers to understand fully the common dietary causes of their attacks and learn how to avoid them. The comprehensive list of appetising recipes demonstrates that to stick to a migraine diet is no hardship. The recipes avoid the common food precipitants of migraine, but it must be recognised that there are still those few unlucky folk whose attacks are sparked off by other foods not considered here. However, for these few the offending food will come to light when several migraine Attack Forms (see Appendix II) have been completed and studied. These sufferers will need to adjust their diet individually, but having learnt the lessons from this book they will find the task of constructing a person-alised diet easy enough.

KATHARINA DALTON, 1981
London W1

Author's Preface

MIGRAINE is one of the oldest known diseases and yet there is still no specific cure. It brings misery to many thousands of people and can be so incapacitating as to disrupt employment and social life. Furthermore, many non-sufferers regard migraine as merely a rather grand name for a headache, so that sufferers are often treated as malingerers and hypochondriacs.

But the pain of migraine is very real indeed and the visual disturbances and constant vomiting or nausea cause much distress to those who experience them. The usual medical treatment consists of strong painkillers and ergotamine derivatives, with rest in a darkened room until the attack subsides. Ergotamine, however, can cause unpleasant side-effects when taken frequently or in too high a dosage – not least of these are recurring throbbing headaches! So migraine sufferers often find they are caught up in a vicious circle.

I hope to show in this book that a great deal of self-help can be achieved by every sufferer, principally by strict attention to diet, eliminating certain foods, and eating regularly every 3 to 5 hours.

For many years I did not realise that my terrible headaches were in fact migraine attacks. Then one day a friend, who suffered from migraine, saw me during one of my 'headaches' and explained to me that I was experiencing a full-blown migraine attack. I visited my local doctor and after much questioning he agreed that I had migraine and prescribed MIGRIL tablets (an ergotamine derivative). These certainly shortened the duration of my attacks considerably, but they did nothing to stop their frequency. And, as you are only allowed to take so many ergotamine tablets in a week, I sometimes found I had to suffer a complete attack without them.

Some time later I consulted Dr Katharina Dalton, who suggested that I should come off the contraceptive pill. This dramatically reduced the frequency and length of my attacks, but I was still having attacks far too often for comfort, and both my work and social life were being continually disrupted. It was then that Dr Dalton suggested that certain foods might be precipitating the migraine attacks. It had never occurred to me that I might be allergic to certain foods and I didn't really believe this could be so. I had never noticed any pattern of attacks connected with what I ate. I had long been an ardent follower of the health foods movement and I ate well-balanced, nutritious meals with plenty of fresh fruit and vegetables.

However I had nothing to lose, so I agreed to keep migraine Attack Forms (copies in Appendix II) which recorded the foods and beverages I had consumed throughout the 48 hours previous to an attack. They also reported the times I had taken food and drink. It soon became apparent that red wine and cheese were the principal culprits, followed by chocolate and tinned frozen orange juice. Later I added pork and pork products to my personal list of offenders. These had been harder to detect since I found I could eat small amounts with no problem, but if I had pork for several meals or days running, then it appeared to have a cumulative effect.

It was a great blow to find that I was allergic to some of my favourite foods, which previously I had eaten

12

frequently, but I did find that when I excluded them from my diet I could go for long periods without an attack.

Any migraine attacks I have now are usually related to going without food for 5 hours (daytime) or 13 hours (overnight) and therefore partially self-induced. I still find it very hard to stick to the strict routine of eating every 3 to 5 hours.

Over the years I have learned to cope with my disability and have found that there are still many delicious things to eat which do not include cheese, chocolate, red wine or citrus fruit – the foods which most often precipitate migraine. In this book I hope to share with you everything that has helped me control my attacks and to give you some idea of the wide variety of dishes for breakfast, lunch and dinner which can be made without including these foods. I hope, too, that you will experiment for yourself with new dishes and that you will fill in the Attack Forms meticulously so that you can work out your own personal diet plan.

JOSIE A. WENTWORTH

Part I

Migraine – the Facts

1

What is Migraine?

ROUGHLY half the population rarely or never suffers from headaches, but of the half that does, approximately 1 in 5 are migraine sufferers, making a total incidence of migraine-sufferers a staggering 8 to 10 per cent of the general population – perhaps 6 million sufferers in Britain alone.

Many people will ask what is the difference between a headache and migraine? Migraine is a vascular headache which causes intense throbbing pain on one side of the head (either right or left) and is accompanied by nausea, vomiting, biliousness and/or visual disorders. The sufferer is severely debilitated and cannot continue his or her normal routine. The attacks occur at intervals and ordinary painkiller tablets give little or no relief.

On the other hand, a tension headache is a dull persistent pain often likened to a heavy weight or a tight band around the head. It is not accompanied by nausea and vomiting or visual disorders. The pain is produced by tension and pressure in the muscles of the neck and head, caused by stress and worry. Tension headaches can be chronic and be present more or less continuously, whereas migraine comes and goes in a definite attack. However, it is possible to suffer from both tension headaches *and* migraine.

There are two types of migraine, common and

classical. Twice as many people suffer from common migraine as from classical migraine, although sufferers of frequent attacks of common migraine will often have occasional attacks of the classical type.

Common migraine is a unilateral headache accompanied by nausea and/or vomiting. In classical migraine these symptoms are preceded by warning signs called an 'aura'. The signs are usually visual and are followed by acute headache pain approximately 20 minutes later. These visual disturbances can be in the form of zig-zag lines, coloured shapes or flashing lights. The vision may become blurred and the ability to focus on objects impaired. In some cases, part of the sufferer's field of vision is blotted out completely. In very rare instances, there is temporary paralysis of a limb or even half the body.

Other warning signs include a feeling of extra well-being, or a sense of remoteness; sudden excess energy; nausea; extreme hunger or thirst. With these non-visual warning signs the period between the 'aura' and the onset of the headache pain may be much longer than the usual 20 minutes.

What Happens in a Classical Migraine Attack?

Some hours or perhaps only minutes before the onset of an attack, warning signs are experienced. These could include any of the following symptoms:

Visual disturbances: double vision, difficulty in focusing, temporary partial blindness, dazzling coloured lights, spots, lines or zig-zags
Numbness, tingling sensation, dizziness, trembling, weakness
Hallucinations

18

Nausea, vomiting
Sensitivity to noise or light
Depression, irritability, tension
Exaggerated well-being, alterations in mood and
    outlook
Unusual hunger
Excitability and talkativeness
Speech difficulties
Pains in neck and shoulders
Blotchy patches on skin, or rashes
Inflamed scalp
Unusual pallor, especially in children
Noticeable increase in weight
Swelling of fingers, waist or breasts
Increase in frequency or volume of urination
Excessive thirst

These signs are all associated with the biochemical
changes which occur at the onset of a migraine attack.
Latest research indicates that migraine is caused by a
malfunction of vaso-active amine metabolism, allowing
the release of vaso-dilating amines which cause the blood
vessels to dilate or expand. Vaso-active amines affect
the size of blood vessels and can cause them either to
constrict or to dilate. There are a vast number of
different vaso-active amines implicated in the cause of
migraine, and these amines are all broken down or
metabolised in the body by a group of enzymes called
monoamine oxidase enzymes. Research has led us to
believe that migraine sufferers have some localised
deficiency of monoamine oxidase enzymes, which
interferes with their ability to metabolise vaso-active
amines.

Migraine, therefore, is a biochemical disorder and
changes occur in the affected blood vessels during an

19

attack. It tends to run in families: people are born with a predisposition to migraine, and have a constitutional tendency for their blood vessels to react abnormally to certain stimuli. Vaso-active amines, which are contained in many of the foods we eat every day, can act as a stimulus and cause constriction of large arteries and veins and dilation of smaller arteries and arterioles.

During the first phase of a migraine there is a narrowing of the branches of the carotid blood vessels. This affects the blood vessels on both sides of the head, not just those on the side which will eventually become painful. The retinal vessels on both sides of the head also narrow, and this can be confirmed by examination of the eyes with an ophthalmoscope. In fact, the blood flow in the internal carotid may be reduced to half its previous level.

In the next stage of an attack, the blood vessels on the side of the head where the pain soon develops become

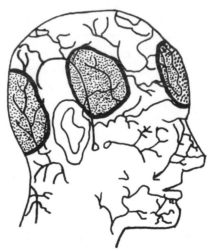

The arteries of the scalp, branches of the external carotid artery. (The sites of pain in migraine are indicated by the shaded areas.)

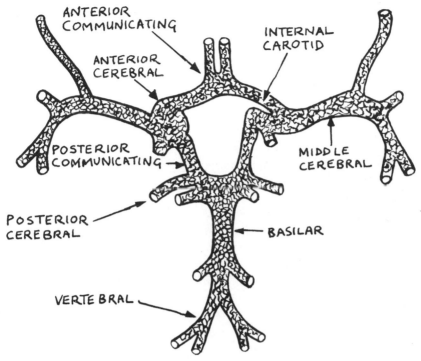

Arteries at the base of the brain, the circle of Willis.

enlarged and start to throb. The pain affects primarily the eye and temple, the side of the head and the back of the neck, but it can spread up from the neck to the top of the head or down into the shoulder of the side affected. The pain is intense and throbs continuously; any slight noise, bright light or movement, especially when bending down, will aggravate it. Sometimes there are stabbing and shooting pains. It is at this stage that the sufferer is forced to lie down in some dark place, with his head buried in a pillow.

During an attack the sufferer looks very pale and ill. He often feels cold and shivery, and has cold hands and

21

feet. In spite of this, his head is very hot. The fact that the blood flow is increased in the painful area could account for the considerable heat given off by the head. It is strange, however, that the face remains white and pale, not flushed, and that the sufferer actually feels cold. The most likely explanation for this is that probably the blood is being pumped to the deeper tissues so that despite the fact that more blood is flowing through the arteries it is not reaching the skin.

The skin of the whole head may now be extremely painful to touch and this condition could last for several days after the attack proper is over. The skin is inflamed and the whole area becomes very sore and hot. Sometimes this condition can *precede* an attack.

An attack can last for an hour, several hours, or even several days. It is not unknown for sufferers eventually to fall asleep from sheer exhaustion only to find the intolerable pain still there when they awake.

For anyone who has not endured a migraine attack, it is hard to imagine the agony that takes place. The nearest I can get to explaining it is to ask you to imagine the worst sea sickness you have ever experienced and to add to that a throbbing headache which is so bad you cannot move, and you will have some idea of how a sufferer feels in an acute attack.

More women than men suffer from migraine. Figures in a recent survey give a ratio of 7 females to 4 males. The possible reasons for this are discussed in Chapter 9.

Men suffer more headaches and migraine attacks between the ages of 15 and 54, after which the incidence tends to decline. Women are not so lucky. They suffer more attacks than men in the age group 15 to 34, and between the ages of 35 to 54 attacks increase even more, declining only marginally after the age of 55.

Migraine attacks usually start in the early teens – between 13 and 14. This could be due to hormonal changes taking place, which can be a sensitising factor affecting amine metabolism. Some women only experience migraine when they have been on the contraceptive pill and here we have very definite evidence of the link between hormone balance and migraine.

Three quarters of a million children under the age of 10 suffer from migraine but this often goes undetected because it usually takes the form of abdominal migraine, causing stomach pains and biliousness accompanied by vomiting, but not necessarily by headache. As children have upset stomachs for many different reasons, it is only when the child grows up and starts to have migraine attacks with head pain, nausea and vomiting etc., that it is, in retrospect, possible to see that those childhood bilious attacks were really migraine. Recent research shows that many children start their attacks before the age of 5 and in these cases they are invariably caused by the same food allergies that affect their parents, or by long intervals *without* food. However, where food is involved, the time lapse between ingesting the food and the onset of the attack is much shorter with children than with adults. Therefore mother and daughter could eat the same food and the daughter might start vomiting immediately or within a few hours, while the mother's migraine might not start for 12 to 48 hours, or more.

2

Triggers Precipitating Migraine

ALTHOUGH extensive research has already been done and is still continuing, the actual cause of the migraine attack is still not proven. However, research does show that certain things will trigger migraine in susceptible individuals. The Migraine Trust (see Appendix I) lists more than 30 such triggers; but when these are examined carefully they can be combined within 6 major categories:

1 Food sensitivity/allergy
2 Hypoglycaemia/low blood sugar
3 Tension and stress
4 Water retention
5 Depression
6 Menstruation and the contraceptive pill

The unfortunate thing is that a large number of sufferers are quite unaware of all the things which can trigger their migraines. For a long time doctors have told their patients that migraine is caused by stress and tension; and so many sufferers have always thought their attacks to be a result of emotional stress, without ever becoming aware of the real culprit.

Even the 6 categories of triggers, listed above, can be reduced. Tension, stress and depression can inhibit appetite so that sufferers may not eat; their blood sugar will drop and they will experience hypoglycaemic reactions which they will not recognise as such. In women, water retention is frequently caused by an imbalance of hormones during the menstrual cycle, making the sufferer feel fat and bloated, and often depressed. When a woman feels like this, she does not want to eat. It is highly likely that a woman suffering from water retention will lose or restrict her appetite, eat less and then suffer low blood sugar reactions. And, as every woman knows, menstruation can cause tension and depression as well as water retention and loss of appetite. The Pill can have the same effect, but with the added hazard that it can result in weight gain. A woman putting on weight feels depressed and tries to slim, stops eating and consequently suffers from low blood sugar symptoms.

Foods which appear to precipitate migraine are those which contain vaso-active amines. Tyramine, phenylethylamine, histamine, isoamylamine, octopamine, synephrine and 5-hydroxytryptamine are just some of the offending amines. However, some people may react to only one or two of these amines while others, fortunately very few, will be sensitive to them all. Some sufferers will not be able to tolerate even a slight trace of any of these amines, while others may be able to cope with them all in small amounts.

To give you an idea of the effect of these amines in susceptible individuals: normally ingesting 3 mg of phenylethylamine will induce a migraine; 10 mg of tyramine will produce a migraine type of reaction and 100 mg will give a severe migraine attack; as will only 8 mg histamine. As much as 1.5 mg per gramme (42 mg per ounce) of tyramine has been found in some cheeses.

Recent research suggests that in those with a biochemical defect in amine metabolism, food allergy may be the final precipitating factor in a migraine attack. However, sensitising factors have usually been present at an earlier stage. Fasting (5 hours without food daytime; 13 hours overnight) may be one such sensitising factor. Others are: the changing levels of menstrual hormones; stress, causing alteration in adrenal hormone levels; lack of sleep and alteration of body rhythms.

Dr Katharina Dalton has done much work in migraine research and, in 1975, she conducted a survey on the hormonal aspects of migraine in 2,000 female sufferers. Everyone involved in the survey completed an Attack Form which, as well as requesting information about the patient's menstrual cycle, asked for a complete list of the foods eaten during the 24 hours immediately before the onset of an attack and at what time the food was eaten. Although this survey had been primarily concerned with hormonal questions, when the Attack Forms were analysed it was found that 95% of the participants had either ingested foods containing vaso-active amines – cheese, chocolate, citrus fruits and alcohol – or had low blood sugar due to the fasting prior to their attack. Fasting was defined as taking no food for 5 hours in daytime or 13 hours overnight.

The final question on the Attack Form asked: 'What do you think caused this attack?' Only 14% mentioned food at all and only 2% thought that fasting could have been responsible: whereas stress, worry and tension were frequently cited. Even when the evidence of food sensitivity was put before the patients, many could not accept it as the cause.

A migraine-sufferer myself, I also did not think that food could possibly be the cause of my attacks until I systematically tested each suspect food and completed an Attack Form. The enormous number of severe attacks I experienced during those self-imposed trials did more than convince me that eating what had been my favourite foods had in fact amounted to playing with poison.

The whole question of food allergy and low blood sugar is complicated. We must also consider body rhythms and the individual. No two people are alike, but if you monitor your attacks very carefully you will soon find the triggers that relate to you, and your personal tolerance levels.

Let us look at body rhythms. Throughout the day the body is a hive of activity, keeping everything working correctly, supplying and withdrawing chemicals as and when they are needed. The rhythms of these activities affect our moods, energy levels, susceptibility to illness and our reactions to food and drugs. Doctors have long known that many drugs are more effective when taken at certain times. You will have noticed that most prescriptions specify when the pills or medicine are to be taken: in the morning, last thing at night, before or after food. Armed with this knowledge, let us return to food sensitivity or allergy in connection with migraine. It is possible that you will find you can tolerate a particular food at one time but not at another. I know a number of sufferers who can happily drink orange juice for breakfast, but cannot tolerate it in the evening.

Another thing to remember about triggers is that their effect is cumulative. You may be able to cope with one trigger, but add two or three together and it is unlikely that you will escape an attack. For example, a person who has had a stressful day, has skipped lunch, is ravenously hungry and so decides to eat a bar of chocolate, is far more likely to develop a migraine than the same person on a restful day, when he or she has eaten regularly, and decides to have a chocolate at the end of an enjoyable meal.

Stress and tension may increase your sensitivity to certain foods. So too do changes in the hormone balance. A woman may well find that she can tolerate alcohol for most of the month, but that even one glass on the days in the premenstrual period will induce a migraine. The same could be true of cheese; you might find that, as long as you eat small amounts and choose cheeses with low tyramine levels (see Chapter 5), you experience no ill effects. But if you eat cheese when you are upset or worried, or perhaps when you are ovulating or menstruating, the effect will be a bad migraine.

Dr Dalton has kindly agreed to allow me to quote from some of her case histories[*] to help illustrate the problems involved in spotting migraine triggers. Perhaps you will be able to identify with some of the situations in your own life and see for the first time what actually triggered your attack.

Time Lapse

CASE 1   'A 54-year-old male director suspected that dairy foods provoked attacks and he had successfully avoided them for 3 years, until he was tempted to eat some yoghurt. After 24 hours he phoned to tell me that no dire results had befallen him – but a second call the next day informed me that severe migraine had developed after 36 hours.'

It can take anything from 12 to 48 hours after eating an offending food for a migraine to develop.

Food Sensitivities

The most satisfactory trigger factors to eliminate are in those patients whose attacks result from tyramine

[*]Taken, together with Dr Dalton's comments, from 'Migraine – A Personal View' by Katharina Dalton MRCS, LRCP, *Proceedings of the Royal Society of Medicine*, March 1973. Vol. 66, No. 3, pp. 263–266.

sensitivity, and here one must acknowledge the work of Edda Hanington who, in 1967, demonstrated the link between migraine and the ingestion of tyramine in susceptible individuals. The commonest food containing tyramine is cheese, but as the time interval between ingestion and onset of attack is usually about 20 to 24 hours the cause, too, often passes unrecognised.

CASE 1 'A housewife aged 47 attended with three completed Attack Forms. Together we observed that her migraine had occurred 20 hours after a meal of cheese. Then she suddenly became crestfallen as she recalled that the previous evening she had eaten 4 oz (120 g) of Cheddar cheese for supper when she was alone in the house. At 4 p.m. that afternoon her husband phoned to say that she was having her worst ever migraine.'

Recognition of tyramine sensitivity can alter an individual's life pattern, especially in those whose attacks were previously considered to be of psychological origin.

CASE 2 'A financial executive, aged 37, suffered from occasional attacks while working in a London suburb. His firm then moved him to central London and there he had frequent migraine. This was attributed to the extra responsibility entailed in his work. After a year he returned to his former office in the suburbs where the attacks were less severe. It was only when thought was given to the possibility of an offending food that it was appreciated that in central London he often had time for only a quick pub lunch of a cheese sandwich and beer whereas in the local office there was time for a proper meal. Now he can pinpoint attacks, which are always due to a dietary indiscretion.'

29

Tyramine Sensitivity Diminishes During Pregnancy

CASE 1 'A mother aged 34 recognised that attacks were precipitated by chocolate, wine and cheese and was delighted to find that after the first trimester of her second pregnancy she could eat these foods with impunity. As she had planned to limit her family to two she indulged in the best of wines and the most expensive chocolates for the duration of this pregnancy.'

Hypoglycaemia

There are those whose attacks are precipitated by long intervals without food or preceded by an unprovoked and insatiable hunger. Inaccurately, these are usually referred to as 'hypoglycaemic' although their fasting blood sugar is usually no lower than controls, and insulin-induced hypoglycaemia in a diabetic only rarely provokes an attack of migraine. It seems that in these individuals there is a metabolic abnormality with insulin resistance[*] and a defect in breakdown of liver glycogen.[†] Many who claim that attacks are precipitated by fatigue are included in this group. They include those who miss a meal when working overtime, the ones who continue gardening until the last glimmer of light has gone and those who are determined to finish their decorating before stopping for a meal. Attacks among those

[*]Hockaday, J. M., Williamson, D. H., Alberti, K. G. H. M., 'Effects of Intravenous Glucose on some Blood Metabolites & Hormones in Migrainous Subjects', *Background to Migraine*, Cumings, J. N., Editor, Wm Heinemann Medical Books, London 1973.
[†]Pearce, J., Ron, M. A., de Silva, K. L., 'Further Studies of Carbohydrate Metabolism in Migraine', *Background to Migraine*, Cumings, J. N., Editor, Wm Heinemann Medical Books, London 1973.

following a low carbohydrate diet and during religious fasts are precipitated by hypoglycaemia. Those who are unable to sleep on at weekends because they wake up with an attack should consider the possibility of hypoglycaemia, and try the effect of a late night snack. Hypoglycaemia is more common during the days before menstruation and on the postcoital day. The possibility exists that fasting as a cause may be masked by an apparently obvious psychological precipitant (Case 1 below), or by fatigue and tension (Case 2 below).

CASE 1 'A housewife aged 42 had a light fish supper on Friday at 7 p.m. On Saturday she rose at 7 a.m., had no breakfast, and went shopping from 8 to 10 a.m. Then a hurried change for her son's wedding, leaving home at 11.30 a.m. Severe migraine with vomiting developed at 2.30 p.m. after $18\frac{1}{2}$ hours without food.'

CASE 2 'A woman aged 45, mother of three children, part-time clerk. Attacks occurred on Thursday. She attributed the attacks to fatigue and tension, as, after leaving work at midday on Thursday, she would drive 12 miles to her favourite supermarket, buy a week's shopping, then drive home in time to pick up her daughter from school and take her to a weekly dancing lesson. Admittedly it was a tight schedule, accompanied by fear that traffic delays might prevent her completing it, but it was noticed that apart from early morning tea and mid-morning coffee she had no food until 4.30 p.m. The previous evening meal was at 9 p.m., so she went 19 hours without food, taking only drinks.'

It is very tempting if you are worried or upset to sit down and have a glass of brandy to calm you down, or a gin and tonic to give you a lift. In fact, more often than not, friends and relations will suggest it as instant help. But beware – your body may react to it like poison because it is already working overtime to cope with the stress and it does not have available the chemicals to break down and assimilate the alcohol. Again, if you are working on a very tight schedule and find you have missed lunch, think twice before gobbling that innocent bar of chocolate – you could be sticking a knife into yourself!

3

Low Blood Sugar

IN THE LAST chapter we discussed migraine triggers and you will perhaps have noticed that all triggers are greatly increased in effect by low blood sugar levels.

The majority of migraine sufferers have a tendency to low blood sugar which is probably inherited. So what is low blood sugar (hypoglycaemia)? It is the opposite of diabetes – the patient produces too much insulin. The exact amount of over-production of insulin varies enormously from person to person, and although in severe cases hyperinsulin can be fatal, we are now concerned with the majority of cases where the over-production of insulin as insulin resistance, although way above normal and sufficient to produce some very unpleasant symptoms, is nowhere near danger level.

The symptoms of severe insulin shock are feelings of lightheadedness, faintness, palpitations of the heart and a cold sweat. The person complains of a severe headache and often has double vision. He or she may begin to tremble and become unsteady on their feet. In spite of feeling famished the patient is likely to vomit any food he has taken to relieve his hunger or, at best, is overcome with waves of nausea. If the blood sugar continues to fall the patient will faint. (Have you noticed how many of these symptoms are the same as those experienced in the 'aura' stage preceding a migraine attack?)

33

Normally, insulin is secreted at frequent intervals in response to the metabolic demand but that is all, whereas the diabetic's secretion of insulin is scanty and insufficient for the body's needs. The hypoglycaemic, on the other hand, receives a continuous outpouring of insulin.

Blood sugar is the fuel for every cell in the body. But, while the other cells derive nourishment from other sources, the brain is nourished by the glucose in the blood. So, as blood sugar or glucose levels drop, depression and a state of panic or nervous tension and anxiety result. The brain is literally being starved and is panicking in an attempt to keep itself functioning.

Hypoglycaemia cannot be cured or controlled by a miracle drug, but it can be controlled by adherence to a special diet. This places the responsibility for controlling the condition entirely with the patient. This is not easy, as it means sacrificing many of the self-indulgences previously considered relatively harmless.

Before we discuss the diet in greater detail, it is important to understand what happens when food is ingested by a hypoglycaemic person. In a hypoglycaemic, too much insulin is secreted in response to metabolic demand. The liver uses the insulin and stores too much sugar in the cells, leaving insufficient sugar circulating in the blood. The net result of eating a meal can therefore be a further drop in blood sugar.

You might think that the answer is to add more sugar to your diet. Unfortunately, eating more sugar only aggravates the problem because ingesting it acts as a direct stimulant to the body to produce more insulin and the hypoglycaemic is back to square one. Coffee, or rather the caffeine contained in it, is one of many stimulants to the adrenal which indirectly, but nevertheless surely, instigates a chain reaction which ends up with the production of more insulin.

34

If you are prone to waking up in the morning with a migraine or if you find that a migraine inevitably develops when you have indulged in a Sunday morning lie-in, low blood sugar may be responsible. If the nausea accompanying the migraine is not too severe and you can force yourself to have a hearty breakfast, you may find this is sufficient to disperse the attack. But it is a strong-willed person who can force himself to eat a high protein breakfast without coffee or strong tea, when he feels like throwing up. The temptation is to bury one's head in the pillows and try to escape the pain in further sleep. But if you do so, you are likely to be in for a day-long attack.

I have just mentioned the sort of breakfast that should be aimed for; this is indicative of the whole diet that should be adopted if you suspect you suffer from low blood sugar. Incidentally, you can have no fear of adopting such a diet whether your blood sugar is low or normal, for it can do you no harm.

The key to this diet is little and often with high protein and a relatively high fat content (fat helps to depress the activity of the islands of Langerhans, the glands which produce insulin). Obviously, the fat content should be watched and when you have controlled your condition it should be reduced.

It has been suggested that the action of vaso-active amines is increased if they are ingested with fat. Personally, I try to eliminate as many animal fats as possible from my diet, cooking with vegetable or sunflower oil only. Fat can be easily and safely added to the diet in the form of a salad dressing made with a few teaspoonfuls of sunflower oil mixed with a little cider vinegar. Toss your daily salad in this delicious dressing and forget about any other fat. However, if you are on a fat-free diet or have a heart condition, do please consult your doctor before making any change in your diet.

The idea is to eat frequent small meals high in protein, low in easily absorbable carbohydrates. Sugar should be excluded wherever possible if not completely, as should caffeine. You should aim to eat a protein snack at least every 4 hours and to go no longer than 12 hours overnight without food. This diet will not cause an increase in weight because you do not eat *more* food, you simply eat *more frequently*. You will find that protein foods are more satisfying than carbohydrates and therefore you will not want so much.

Low blood sugar sufferers should aim for a diet which gives 80 protein grammes per day to start with. Table 1 at the end of this chapter lists protein contents of principal foods. As the blood sugar levels stabilise you may find that you can manage with less protein, but as everyone has a different metabolism you must find your own levels.

A suitable diet for a low blood sugar sufferer would be on the following lines:

On Waking, Before Arising:

4 fl. oz (120 ml) of pineapple juice

1 cup of decaffeinated coffee (unsweetened, if possible, or sweetened with ½ teaspoonful honey)

1 digestive biscuit

Breakfast:

Fresh pear/slice fresh pineapple/apple/peach/apricot

2 poached eggs on 1 slice wholemeal toast and butter *or* 3 oz (90 g) poached or grilled fish plus 1 slice wholemeal bread (a vegetable such as cabbage, cucumber or celery could be substituted for the wholemeal bread)

36

Mid-morning:

2 oz (60 g) cottage cheese with 1 wholemeal biscuit, *or* 1 chicken drumstick

4 fl. oz (120 ml) of apple juice *or* tisane *or* decaffeinated coffee

Lunch:

3 or 4 oz (90–120 g) fish/meat/2 eggs (not eggs if they have been eaten for breakfast)

Salad with French dressing *or* small helping vegetables (not too much potato but do not cut out completely unless substituting with 1 slice wholemeal bread)

Mid-afternoon (Tea):

2 oz (60 g) cottage cheese plus 1 wholemeal biscuit *or* standard carton yoghurt (if tolerated) *or* 8 fl. oz (240 ml) milk or milk-shake plus 1 wholemeal biscuit *or* 2 oz (60 g) sardines on toast

Dinner:

4 fl. oz (120 ml) apple juice

Soup

3 or 4 oz (90–120 g) meat/fish/poultry plus vegetables

1 slice wholemeal bread

After Dinner:

(Every 2 to 3 hours before retiring)

4 fl. oz (120 ml) milk *or* 2 oz (60 g) nuts *or* 2 oz (60 g) cottage cheese

Obviously this is only a rough guide, to give an idea of what to aim for. Cut down carbohydrates but do *not* cut them out completely. Fresh salads dressed with oil and vinegar (preferably sunflower oil and cider vinegar) can be eaten freely as desired. Out go cakes, pastries, sugar, sweets, puddings and desserts, and in exchange eat plenty of fresh fruit. An adequate amount of fresh fruit, salads and vegetables are important to help you digest the protein.

You may find that after feeling ravenous you can sit down to a high protein meal and, after a few mouthfuls, your appetite suddenly vanishes. This is due to a rapid change in the level of sugar in the blood caused by the activity of digesting the food you are eating. A small spoonful of honey in warm water will make you feel fine in a couple of minutes and you will be able to resume your meal with pleasure. This is also why a sweet or petit-four at the end of a large meal can be beneficial to you and help you to have enough blood sugar to digest your meal. But go easy and remember 'just a little' is your motto.

Then there is the question of exercise. Exercise quickens the metabolic processes of the body. So if you suffer from low blood sugar, exercise will cause your blood sugar to drop faster than the average person's and increase your need for food.

During my research for this book many people kindly sent me details of peculiarities relating to migraine attacks. One I remember very clearly, since it made headlines in several newspapers, reported that 'immoderate sexual indulgence could lead to headaches and migraine'! It went on to tell of a vigorous young man, with a previous history of migraine, who was told by his doctor to slow down his marital transports 3 days after his wedding because of the migraine headaches they were causing. It further reported that these headaches were often accompanied by tremors and sweating. Various possible reasons were given for these attacks, but I believe the most likely explanation was that the exercise involved in sexual intercourse was causing his blood sugar levels to drop, resulting in headaches, migraine and other low blood sugar symptoms. So my advice to you is to make sure you have a good meal before any vigorous lovemaking sessions and if they look like going on *all* night incorporate eating as part of your love play, like suggesting a midnight feast of aphrodisiac foods. You will be amazed at your stamina as long as you ensure you have frequent snacks!

Of course this doesn't just apply to sex. A violent game of squash after work will have the same effect as delaying your evening meal by about 2 hours. I am not advocating that you do not take exercise. Quite the contrary. Exercise is most important for general good health. But it is essential that you realise the effect it has on the metabolism of a low blood sugar sufferer, so that you can adjust your diet accordingly.

Keeping Frequency Charts (see Appendix III) and Attack Forms to show exactly which days you have migraine attacks and at what time they begin, can be invaluable for spotting low blood sugar as a possible cause. Often people will not realise they have been without food for 6 hours or more unless they have kept a record of when food was taken. Fasting or low blood sugar as a trigger precipitating migraine is far more common than is generally realised. Women seem to be more susceptible to low blood sugar than men and especially so in the days during or after menstruation.

The following case histories are taken from *Migraine in General Practice* by Dr Katharina Dalton MRCGP and originally appeared in *The Journal of the Royal College of General Practitioners, 1973* (23,97). They illustrate the way fasting can precipitate migraine attacks.

PATIENT 1 'This was a single, 27-year-old female secretary. The attacks were at fortnightly intervals originally on Tuesdays, but later on Thursdays. Further questioning as to what Tuesday activity had transferred to Thursday, revealed that on Tuesday she went direct from work to her hairdresser, having only had a snack lunch. The migraine developed on her way home at about 20.00 hours. When her favourite hairdresser changed her late night to Thursday the patient changed her appointment. Fasting was the trigger factor.'

PATIENT 2 'This was a male clerk of 42 years, single. The attacks were at weekends and bank holidays, present on rising at 10.00 to 11.00 hours instead of waking with the alarm at 07.30 on working days. These attacks proved to be related to fasting.'

PATIENT 3 'This was a female medical auxiliary, 54 years old. She rose at 07.30 hours on Saturday, had coffee and an Energen biscuit. She was anxious not to gain weight after having stopped smoking. At 12.45 in a restaurant a severe migraine developed before starting a meal.'

PATIENT 4 'This was a male sales representative, of 34 years. Sunday 08.00 hours breakfast of porridge, egg and bacon, toast and coffee. He played 18 holes of golf. No further food or drink was taken until 18.00 hours when he developed a classical migraine.'

The Sunday morning headache is perhaps the best example of fasting migraine. Often the sufferer has had an early evening meal on Saturday night before going out for an evening's entertainment, perhaps a party or a discotheque, and then has a long lie-in on Sunday morning, only to wake with a splitting migraine. The answer to this is to have a late night snack and to put some milk and biscuits by the bed to eat immediately you wake in the morning. When you have eaten something in the morning, by all means turn over, go back to sleep and enjoy a lie-in.

Sometimes an apparently psychological cause for migraine will mask the real culprit, fasting, as demonstrated in the hypoglycaemic cases 1 and 2, described in the previous chapter.

If you think your attack could be due to fasting or low blood sugar, remember that you can easily remedy the situation by eating frequent snacks at 3 to 4 hourly intervals. These snacks can be of non-fattening foods but should be high in protein, and if you divide your total daily calorie allowance into 6 snacks instead of 3 meals, this should not affect your weight.

Low blood sugar is something all migraine sufferers should watch very carefully. We know it can precipitate attacks on its *own*, but it can *also* act as a sensitising factor for food allergies. The following four chapters deal with each of the principal offenders.

TABLE 1
Protein Content of Some Common Foods

The information contained in these tables has been compiled from *The Agricultural Handbook No. 8* and *Home and Garden Bulletin No. 72*, issued by the USA Department of Agriculture, Washington D.C.

When the foods were analysed they were weighed in grammes, so the gramme weight in the first column is the exact weight. An approximate imperial measure has been given in the second column for your easy reference. A conversion factor of 28.35 grammes to the ounce has been used and then the figure rounded up or down to give a familiar imperial measure. (In the recipe section of this book, and elsewhere, the convenient conversion factor of 30 grammes to 1 ounce has been used.)

FOOD	WEIGHT IN GRAMMES	APPROX. IMPERIAL MEASURE	PROTEIN GRAMMES
Bread and Cereals			
Bread			
White, 20 slices	454	1 lb loaf	39
Wholewheat	454	1 lb loaf	48
Wholewheat	23	1 slice	2
Macaroni, cooked	140	5 oz	5

Noodles	160	5½ oz	7
Oatmeal, rolled oats	236	8¼ oz	5
Pancakes, 4 in/10 cm diam. wheat	108	4 pancakes	7
Rice			
Brown	208	7¼ oz	15
White	191	6¾ oz	14
Spaghetti, with meat sauce	250	8¾ oz	13
Wheatgerm	104	3½ oz	26
Wholewheat flour	120	4 oz	13
White flour	110	4 oz	12
Dairy Products			
Buttermilk, cultured	246	8 fl. oz	9
Cheese			
Cottage	225	8 fl. oz	38
Cream	28	1 oz	2
Cream, double	120	4 fl. oz	2
Eggs			
Boiled or poached	100	2 eggs	12
Scrambled, omelette or fried	128	2 eggs	13
Yolks only	34	2	6
Milk			
Cows, skimmed	984	32 fl. oz	36

TABLE 1 *continued*

FOOD	WEIGHT IN GRAMMES	APPROX. IMPERIAL MEASURE	PROTEIN GRAMMES
Cows, whole	976	32 fl. oz	32
Evaporated, undiluted	252	8 fl. oz	16
Powdered, whole	103	8 fl. oz	27
Yoghurt, of partially skimmed milk	250	8 fl. oz	8
Fish			
Cod			
Grilled	100	$3\frac{1}{2}$ oz	28
Fishcakes	100	2 small	15
Fish fingers	112	5 fingers	19
Haddock, fried	85	3 oz	16
Halibut, grilled	100	$3\frac{1}{2}$ oz	26
Herring, kippered	100	1 small	22
Salmon, canned	85	3 oz	17
Sardines, canned	85	3 oz	22
Tuna, canned	85	3 oz	25

Meat, Offal and Poultry, Cooked

Beef			
Chuck, pot roast	3 oz	85	23
Corned, canned	3 oz	85	12
Roast	3 oz	85	16
Steak, braising, lean	3 oz	85	24
Steak, sirloin	3 oz	85	20
Stew with vegetables	8 fl. oz	235	15
Beefburger	3 oz	85	21
Chicken			
Fried	3 oz	85	25
Grilled	3 oz	85	23
Livers, fried	3 medium	100	22
Roast	3½ oz	100	25
Duck, roast	3½ oz	100	16
Lamb			
Braised shoulder of	3 oz	85	18
Chop	4 oz	115	24
Roast leg of	3 oz	86	20
Offal			
Brains, beef, calves, sheep	3½ oz	100	10
Heart, braised	3 oz	85	26
Kidney, braised	3½ oz	100	33

45

TABLE 1 *continued*

FOOD	WEIGHT IN GRAMMES	APPROX. IMPERIAL MEASURE	PROTEIN GRAMMES
Liver, calves 1 large slice	100	$3\frac{1}{2}$ oz	29
Liver, lambs, 2 slices	100	$3\frac{1}{2}$ oz	32
Liver, ox, fried	100	$3\frac{1}{2}$ oz	26
Sweetbreads, calves, braised	100	$3\frac{1}{2}$ oz	32
Tongue, beef	85	3 oz	18
Turkey, roast	100	$3\frac{1}{2}$ oz	27
Veal			
Cutlet, grilled	85	3 oz	23
Roast	85	3 oz	23
Nuts and Seeds			
Almonds, roasted and salted	70	$2\frac{1}{2}$ oz	13
Brazils, unsalted	70	$2\frac{1}{2}$ oz	10
Cashews, unsalted	70	$2\frac{1}{2}$ oz	12
Peanut butter			
Commercial	50	$1\frac{3}{4}$ oz	12
Natural	50	$1\frac{3}{4}$ oz	13
Peanuts, roasted	50	$1\frac{3}{4}$ oz	13
Sesame seeds, raw	50	$1\frac{3}{4}$ oz	9

Sunflower seeds, raw	50	$1\frac{3}{4}$ oz	12
Walnuts, raw	50	$1\frac{3}{4}$ oz	7
Soups, Canned			
Chicken or turkey	250	8 fl. oz	4
Consommé	240	8 fl. oz	5
Cream soups	255	8 fl. oz	7
Split pea	250	8 fl. oz	8
Supplementary Foods			
Brewer's yeast, powdered	33	$1\frac{1}{4}$ oz	13
Dessicated liver, defatted	37	$1\frac{1}{4}$ oz	28
Vegetables			
Artichoke, globe	100	1 large	2
Dandelion greens, steamed	180	$6\frac{1}{4}$ oz	5
Kale, steamed	110	$3\frac{3}{4}$ oz	4
Lentils	200	7 oz	15
Peas			
Fresh or frozen, steamed	100	$3\frac{1}{2}$ oz	5
Split, cooked	100	$3\frac{1}{2}$ oz	8
Pepper, green, stuffed with minced beef	150	$5\frac{1}{4}$ oz	19
Soybeans	200	7 oz	22
Spinach, steamed	100	$3\frac{1}{2}$ oz	3

4

Chocolate

CHOCOLATE is the food most commonly suspected by migraine sufferers as being the cause of their attacks. Perhaps this is because chocolate is often associated with a treat or pleasure and it tends to be easier to remember when you ate some. A survey of 500 migraine sufferers who could always relate their attacks to dietary factors showed that 75% cited chocolate as the prime precipitant.

Chocolate contains many different amines but, strangely enough, it does not contain tyramine, the amine which first aroused researchers' suspicions and which is found in such large quantities in cheese. It is the amine 2-phenylethylamine which is the prime offender in chocolate. This amine, incidentally, is also found in substantial quantities in some cheeses and wines. It is interesting and useful to note which foods contain which amines, because a sufferer may be allergic to tyramine and not to 2-phenylethylamine; so he could eat chocolate with no ill effect, but could not touch cheese, and vice versa.

Bitter and plain chocolate have higher levels of 2-phenylethylamine than milk chocolate and white chocolate. The fermentation and maturation of the cocoa bean greatly increase the amine content and the roasting of the fermented beans causes a seven-fold increase in phenylethylamine concentration. Unfortunately, chocolate just wouldn't taste like chocolate if it was made from unfermented fresh cocoa beans! Fermentation and roasting are essential parts of the processing of cocoa products.

In tests, 3 mg of 2-phenylethylamine have induced headaches in susceptible individuals. The reaction can vary from person to person; some people may need to ingest far less to get a reaction while others may be able to tolerate a higher level. There is approximately 3 mg of 2-phenylethylamine in a 2-oz (60 g) bar of chocolate. Of course this will vary from brand to brand depending on the concentration of cocoa.

As I explained in Chapter 2, there are usually sensitising factors at work before a trigger food is ingested. The most likely sensitising factors operating when chocolate is eaten are fasting (low blood sugar) and anxiety or stress. How many of us have been on a shopping spree, not stopped for lunch and then gobbled a bar of chocolate in the car or on the bus home; or have had a rush on at the office so that we skip lunch, feel famished by mid-afternoon and so grab a bar of chocolate to munch with our afternoon cup of tea? Everyone knows that there is a temptation to eat sweets when one is under stress. How many lovers' quarrels or matrimonial upsets are made up with a peace-offering of a box of chocolates, and how many of the recipients later develop a migraine which they automatically blame on the stress caused by the quarrel and never dream that it could be the chocolates?

I know of the case of a woman who suffered from premenstrual tension and always became very depressed and tearful the few days before her period. Her husband was very understanding and did everything he could to cheer her up. He made a particular point of bringing her a beautiful box of luxury chocolates at this time each month. She was very touched by his gesture and felt guilty the next day when she had a migraine. It was only when she was being treated for her migraine attacks and started to eliminate suspect foods from her diet that she thought about the chocolates. She asked her husband if he would bring her flowers instead of chocolates for a while. Miraculously her migraine disappeared. Here we have a classic case of hormonal changes acting as a sensitising factor, causing a stress situation (another sensitiser) and the ingestion of chocolate as the final precipitant of the migraine attack.

Cutting chocolate out of the diet is not easy. There is little else one can substitute for it. The best alternative is the carob pod, also known as the locust-bean. It has a chocolate-like flavour and can be used in cooking for flavouring cakes and desserts. It comes from a tree with glossy dark green leaves which grows all over the world. The best variety has a long flat pod, anything from 3 to 12 inches long, which is dried to make carob powder and other products. The dried pod is brown in colour, like chocolate. The chocolate flavour of carob becomes more pronounced when the pod is ground and even more so when it is cooked.

Although nowadays carob is a speciality food found primarily in health food stores and delicatessens, it has been eaten for thousands of years. It is highly nutritious and is sometimes called St John's Bread because it was believed to have been the food which sustained John the Baptist in the Wilderness.

Unlike cocoa, carob does not have a bitter taste. It contains 46% natural sugar while cocoa only has 5.5%, so it does not need masses of refined sugar added to make it palatable. In spite of carob's sweetness it contains far fewer calories than cocoa, only 177 calories per 100 grammes ($3\frac{1}{2}$ oz approx.) against the 295 calories per 100 grammes in chocolate. Carob is in fact an ideal substitute for chocolate for anyone who is slimming. Not only is it much lower in calories, it also contains less than 1% fat, while cocoa contains 23.7% fat.

Carob can be used in almost all recipes which call for cocoa. However, you may need to use less sugar on account of its natural sweetness. Carob powder stirred into a glass of milk makes a delicious chocolate-flavoured drink. A selection of dishes using carob is included in the recipes contained in the second half of this book.

On the sweet counter, most confectionery which comes in bars is chocolate-coated even if it is not pure chocolate. It is advisable to stick to nougat, fudge, coconut ice or some of the excellent dried fruit and nut bars available in health food stores.

Coffee essence is a good alternative to chocolate for producing sophisticated desserts, and so is butterscotch flavouring. They can be used as substitutes for chocolate in icings, topping, sauces, and creams.

If you are lucky, you may find you can tolerate small amounts of chocolate provided that there are no other sensitising factors. For example, a mint chocolate following a meal, when the blood sugar is high, may well be tolerated but never grab a bar of chocolate when you are hungry and your blood sugar is low, or when you feel upset and overwrought. It may well turn out to be the final trigger that tips the scale and induces a migraine attack.

5

Cheese

CHEESE is the second of the four main offenders that can precipitate migraine attacks. And how delicious cheese is, the easy nutritious snack, the food which requires no preparation, with its sharp distinctive flavouring for sauces and gratin dishes.

Cheese can be a very difficult food to cut out of your diet. However, as it is the tyramine content of cheese which can cause migraine and this varies from one type of cheese to another, making some more lethal than others, there may be some cheeses you can tolerate.

It is the same action of tyramine which causes problems for people taking monoamine oxidase inhibitor (MAOI) antidepressant drugs. In fact the reactions experienced by patients on these drugs stimulated research into tyramine allergy and the results have been of great help to migraine sufferers. Therefore, people taking MAOI antidepressants will find some useful tips in these pages.

All the blue cheeses are exceptionally high in tyramine, as are most of the hard cheeses. The tyramine content of cheese can vary from one piece to another of the same type and, of course, different types contain different amounts. The amount of tyramine tends to increase the longer the cheese is matured. For example, Caerphilly is ready for eating in only 6 weeks and its tyramine content is relatively less. Therefore, small amounts may be tolerated by some people. Some cheeses contain 2-phenylethylamine as well, making these doubly dangerous.

The cheeses to be avoided (maturation time is given in parentheses): Cheddar (3 months); matured Cheddar (7 months); Stilton (3 months); Danish Blue (3 months); Leicester (3 months); Derby and Sage Derby (2 months); Scottish Red mild (3 months); Irish mild (3 months); Cheshire Red and White (6 weeks); Wensleydale (6 weeks).

Soft cheeses such as Camembert and Brie are relatively young cheeses with lower tyramine content and so may be tolerated in small quantities by some sufferers. Cream cheese and cottage cheese have been found to contain *no* tyramine or 2-phenylethylamine and can therefore be eaten without fear.

In control tests, as little as 6 mg of tyramine taken orally in food causes changes in the body and produces a rise in blood pressure. Usually 10 mg of tyramine needs to be ingested to produce a headache, and 100 mg to give a severe migraine attack. As much as 1.5 mg of tyramine has been found in 1 g of some cheeses (42 mg per ounce). Table 2 shows the tyramine content of some common cheeses. However, it must be remembered that this is not the only amine present in cheese. Many cheeses also contain substantial amounts of 2-phenyl-ethylamine and if you are allergic to both amines the cumulative effect can be disastrous. Table 3 shows the 2-phenylethylamine concentration in some cheeses. You will see that Stilton cheese is high both in tyramine and 2-phenylethylamine, as is Cheddar.

Of course, the levels of both amines will vary from manufacturer to manufacturer and from one batch to another. But it would be wise for any migraine sufferer to avoid Stilton and all blue cheeses as well as Cheddar

TABLE 2
Tyramine Content of some Common Cheeses

TABLE 3
2-Phenylethylamine Content of some Common Cheeses

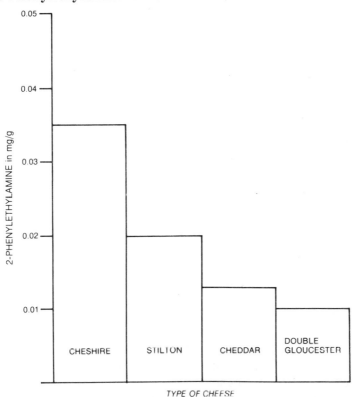

and all hard cheeses. It is possible that a morsel of Camembert eaten at the end of a meal may be tolerated. Some people may even find they can happily eat small portions of Caerphilly or Brie.

Table 2 and Table 3 show the tyramine and 2-phenylethylamine content of *some* cheeses. 'N.Y. State Cheddar' and 'Processed American Cheese' are very similar to our own Cheddar and processed cheese. Many other cheeses do not appear on the charts because accurate data is not readily available, but that does not mean that they do not contain tyramine or 2-phenylethylamine. Migraine sufferers should work on the assumption that all cheeses except cottage and cream cheese contain vaso-active amines. These tables are compiled from authentic medical data.

But remember, migraine is brought about by a combination of triggers. Even if you find you can tolerate small amounts of some cheeses, it would be unwise to eat any cheese (except cottage or cream) when the blood sugar is low – that cheese sandwich at lunch-time or hurried cheese snack is out. No more cheese and wine parties for migraine sufferers – the combination, especially if you drink red wine, will inevitably result in an attack. Do not eat cheese when under stress or in the premenstruum. Some sufferers may find they only have to avoid cheese on certain days of the month in order to be free of their migraine attacks.

For most of us, unfortunately, it means cutting cheese out of our diet altogether with the exception of cream or cottage cheese, both of which seem very bland after the rich, sharp flavours of other cheeses. However, they can be livened up. Try adding finely-chopped garlic to cream cheese and eating it scooped on to fresh sticks of celery. Cottage cheese mashed into a smooth paste with freshly-ground black pepper and chopped olives is a delicious slimming snack. Of course, you can add chopped fruit and nuts to both cottage and cream cheese for an unusual, exotic dish. More ideas for using these cheeses in cooking, and substituting them in dishes which normally require a hard cheese, can be found in the recipe section.

It is surprising how many dishes are enriched with cheese, and if the latter is to be omitted from the diet you must be aware of its hidden presence. Mornay sauces usually contain Cheddar cheese, all gratin dishes are topped with cheese, Parmesan cheese is sprinkled on or included in many traditional Italian pasta dishes. Many cooks include cheese in *Quiche Lorraine*. *Coquille St Jacques* includes a cheese sauce. Traditional French onion soup is served with pieces of toasted cheese floating in it, while traditional minestrone soup is made with Parmesan cheese. Out go cheese biscuits and cheesy cocktail nibbles, cheese soufflés and omelettes. But on the plus side, many, in fact most, cheese-cakes are made with cream or cottage cheese, so there is no need to give up these delicious concoctions.

Cheese was first suspected as a possible precipitant of migraine when it was the main food incriminated in the headache reactions occurring in patients on monoamine oxidase inhibitor drugs. In her book *Migraine* Dr Edda Hanington tells us:

The way in which the monoamine oxidase enzyme entered the migraine field is interesting. In 1952 a new group of drugs was introduced into the treatment of tuberculosis. These drugs acted as inhibitors of monoamine oxidase enzymes in the body; and it was observed that some of the tuberculosis patients who were treated in this way became noticeably more cheerful. Because of this rise in spirits the drug was tried in patients suffering from depression and a marked improvement in some of them was soon apparent. This led to the introduction of monoamine oxidase inhibitor drugs on a large scale for the treatment of depression.

Despite the fact that thousands of patients in the United States were treated with these drugs no adverse reactions to them were reported for three years. Then reports gradually filtered in of severe headaches associated with a rise in blood pressure which occurred in some of the patients on this therapy.

Careful detective work established that these headaches were associated with the eating of certain foods, notably cheese. The substance contained in the cheese that was responsible for these reactions was found to be tyramine, a name derived from *tiri*, the Greek word for cheese. Tyramine is a vaso-active monoamine.

It is normally broken down in the body by the action of monoamine oxidase and exerts action on blood vessels both directly and through releasing nonadrenaline from its stores.

Although cheese was the main food to be incriminated in headache reactions occurring in patients on monoamine oxidase inhibitor drugs, certain other foods were also found to have similar harmful effects. These foods also were subsequently found to contain vaso-active amines. Owing to the inhibition of monoamine oxidase by the monoamine oxidase inhibitor therapy which the patients were receiving, the vaso-active amines in the various foods were not broken down and rendered harmless as they would normally have been and the headache reactions resulted.

The role of monoamine oxidase enzymes in migraine has not yet been determined. It is possible that attacks are associated with a deficiency in part of this enzyme system.

Other foods also found to contain vaso-active amines include: cheese, chocolate, yoghurt, over-ripe bananas, pickled herring, Marmite, and alcoholic beverages – especially Chianti. These foods should be avoided by people on MAOI drugs as well as by migraine-sufferers.

6

Citrus Fruits

CITRUS fruit, the fruit we are always told is so good for us, comes next in the order of offenders in precipitating migraine attacks.

Citrus fruits include the orange, lemon, lime, grapefruit, satsuma, tangerine, mandarin, and the exotic ugli fruit.

When citrus fruits were first suspected as migraine precipitants they were analysed, but the method of analysis failed to confirm the presence of tyramine or octopamine. However, another vaso-active amine was found – synephrine – and a very high concentration of it, as much as 35 mcg per gramme in oranges.

Concentrated fruit juice seems to be the worst offender, especially the concentrated frozen orange juice. Possibly this is because the whole orange, including the rind, is crushed to produce the concentrate. There are usually higher levels of amines in the skins of the fruit than in the fruit itself. Diluted orange squash or cordial will probably be tolerated by many people. The true orange content of the drink is small and the average amount of synephrine present would be between 0.5 to 1.5 mg per litre, whereas in concentrated canned or frozen orange juice this shoots up to anything from 10 to 30 mg per litre. Perhaps it is fortunate that we do not normally drink the concentrated juice of tangerines or

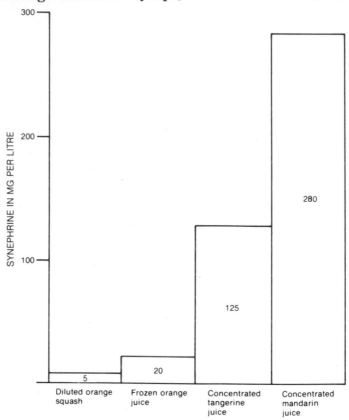

TABLE 4
Average Content of Synephrine in Citrus Fruit Juices

mandarins for they contain far higher levels of synephrine than oranges. Levels of synephrine as high as 125 mg per litre have been recorded in tangerine juice, and in mandarin juice this can be as much as 280 mg per litre.*

I have personally found that a squeeze of lemon or

*Wheaton & Stewart, *Analytical Biochemistry 12*, 585, 1965.

lime juice over a salad or in a cake does no harm and that I can happily drink tea or soft drinks garnished with a thin slice of lemon. This may be because I never eat the slice of lemon, and the amount of juice that actually permeates the drink is so small that the synephrine content is insignificant. I would not, however, contemplate drinking home-made lemonade, made from crushed whole lemons, sugar and water. Lemonade purchased in a bottle is a different matter since it rarely contains any real lemon at all and can therefore be drunk with confidence. This makes a delicious drink when garnished with a slice of cucumber, a sprig of mint and lots of ice cubes. Steer clear of frozen concentrated lemon juice altogether.

Fresh orange juice drunk in the morning seems to be less of a precipitant than if it is taken in the evening. Possibly body rhythms account for this, or there may have been other sensitising factors which happened during the day, so that an orange drink in the evening might just be the final trigger for an attack.

As the offender in citrus fruits and juices is synephrine and not tyramine, there may be many migraine-sufferers who are completely unaffected by these fruits, and who never need to omit them from their diets.

The following fruits can be eaten safely: apples, pears, grapes, pineapples, cherries, gooseberries, blackcurrants, redcurrants, peaches, apricots, figs, plums, lychees, guavas, melon (all types), strawberries, blueberries, bilberries, cranberries and nectarines.

You will notice there are some obvious omissions, and these will be discussed in Chapter 8. Meanwhile, you should be wary of the following, and note your reactions to them carefully: raspberries, loganberries, mulberries, and bananas (especially over-ripe and/or eaten with their skins on).

61

7

And What of Alcohol?

ALCOHOL is the last of the four major migraine precipitants, and is possibly the most difficult to cut out. When we refer to alcohol we are really thinking about alcoholic drinks which contain at most only 50% pure alcohol – the rest of the drink containing many different ingredients to give it a distinctive flavour and colour. So we have to consider not only the effect of the alcohol but also the vaso-active amines present in the other ingredients in alcoholic beverages.

Alcohol itself is a vaso-active substance which dilates the blood vessels and increases the flow of blood to the head. Everyone knows the flushed face of someone who has had too much to drink at a party, or the ruddy complexion of a drunkard. If enough alcohol is imbibed it will give anyone a very bad headache and a nasty hangover, regardless of whether they are migraine-sufferers or not. However, tests have shown that the severity of the headache and hangover depends more on the type of drink that has been consumed than the actual alcohol content. If you drink alcohol alone you can tolerate far more with no ill effects than if you drink it mixed with other flavourings and additives. It is interesting to see that the alcoholic drinks which contain the highest levels of vaso-active amines are the same drinks which will produce the worst hangovers for any drinker.

The actual pure alcohol content of drinks normally available in bars and shops is relatively small, usually less than 50%. Spirits average about 40%; fortified wines (ports, sherries, vermouth etc.,) about 23%; wines 11 to 12%; and beers and lagers often as little as 6 to 7%.

So what to drink and when to drink? It is wise to restrict your drinking habits so that you drink long drinks rather than shorts. Remembering that migraine triggers are cumulative, do not drink alcohol when you are hungry and your blood sugar is low. Beware of cheese snacks and nibbles; cheese and wine parties are out for a migraine-sufferer. You may be able to stand one without the other but there is not much chance that you will be able to consume them together without getting a migraine as a result. As cheese is so frequently served with alcoholic drinks, it is worth remembering that this can be a lethal combination.

For many years I suffered regular migraine attacks on Saturday evenings or Sunday mornings. They caused much misery and played havoc with my social life. All sorts of reasons were suggested for these attacks, including one which really annoyed me; it was intimated that obviously I didn't like week-ends and was using my migraine attacks as an excuse for not going out! When I started to keep migraine Attack Forms the reason for my attacks stood out so plainly I could have kicked myself. It had become a habit of my husband and myself to have a lie-in on Saturday morning, and then to do the week's shopping together, ending up at our local wine bar where we often met friends for lunch. Invariably our meal consisted of a bottle or two of wine (usually red, our preference) and a large helping of French bread, cheese – usually Brie – followed by coffee. By switching to white wine and cold beef or cottage pie I was able to eliminate these migraine attacks completely.

Alcohol is a food similar to sugar in that it provides the

body with calories (energy) but none of the other nutriments essential to health. It is absorbed into the bloodstream as soon as it comes into contact with the walls of the stomach. Alcohol is absorbed more slowly when the stomach is full, so try to restrict drinking to meal-times, or at least try to eat something when you are drinking, or before going out for a drink.

Alcoholic drinks are normally divided up into spirits, wines and beers and we will look at them under these groups. Aperitifs are usually fortified wines or diluted spirits and I have categorised them as 'wines'. Cocktails are more difficult because you must first find out what is in them, so I will treat them separately.

Spirits
A migraine-sufferer should try to avoid spirits whenever possible because of their high alcohol content. However, if you must drink spirits go for gin or vodka and avoid brandy and whisky. Brandy is worse than whisky. The better the brandy (the longer it has matured in the cask) the bigger the hangover and migraine attack. Orange is a favourite accompaniment to both gin and vodka but for amine-sensitive people drinking this is asking for trouble. You may be able to get away with a few gins but adding orange to them may just tip the balance to a full-scale migraine attack. For the same reason beware of liqueurs made with oranges, such as Grand Marnier, Van der Hum or Cointreau. In fact, all liqueurs should be thought about very carefully.

Wines (table wines, aperitifs and fortified wines)
Vaso-active amines which have been found in significant quantities in wines are: tyramine, phenylethylamine and histamine. Fortunately, the amine content varies considerably, depending on the type of wine which you drink. One survey of the histamine content shows a

64

variation of as much as 0 to 30 mg per litre.* The level reported to induce headaches in susceptible persons was found to be 8 mg per litre. Histamine is present in larger quantities in red wine and port than in white wine and sherry.

Vaso-active amines are products of bacterial fermentation and are therefore found in larger quantities in young rather than more mature wines. So Beaujolais Nouveau, for example, is not for migraine-sufferers.

Phenylethylamine has been found in port and Madeira wine, so it is reasonable to suppose it is also present in other red table wines and fortified wines. Red wines generally contain higher levels of vaso-active amines than white wines; this is especially so as regards tyramine. As much as 25 mg per litre of tyramine has been found in Chianti. As you need only 10 mg tyramine or less to induce a migraine, half a bottle of Chianti could give you a very severe attack.

Red wines are made from the fruit pulp and crushed skins of black grapes, which contain high levels of amines, while rosé and white wines use only the fruit pulp without the skins. Studies indicate that wines which have been heated during their preparation contain even higher levels of amines. This would account for the higher levels found in red wines and ports, since these are often heated to extract more colour from the grape skins.

A certain amount of red wine is often added to sweet sherries to give them a greater depth of colour, and this colouring wine has also been heated. This could explain why some people cannot tolerate sweet sherry, but can manage a little dry sherry. However, recent research

*Cugh, C. S., University of California, 'Measurement of Histamine in Californian Wines', *Journal of Agricultural Food Chemistry*, *19*, 241–244, 1971.

shows that *all* sherries, sweet and dry, contain high levels of vaso-active amines of many different types, and should generally be avoided by migraine-sufferers. It is also worth noting that the amines in sherry become more active when heated, so that when used in cooking, sherry can become a very potent migraine precipitant, particularly when used in flambé dishes.

Dry white vermouths and white Martinis are safe to drink. With regard to other aperitifs, I suggest that you try them out to find out what suits you. But remember to avoid ports, sweet sherry and all those aperitifs based on red wines and brandy.

So let us sum up the position regarding wine. Red wines contain higher levels of amines than white wines, so it would be wise to avoid all red wines, especially Chianti. A light white wine would probably be tolerated by most people and I suggest a Hock, Riesling or Moselle. Remember, young wines have a higher amine content, so choose a mature wine. Cheap wines contain more impurities, so it is worth paying for a better quality wine, and anyway you can afford to pay more if you are going to drink less of it!

If you are buying French wines, choose those with the *appellation contrôlée* label. If you are buying German wines, choose a *Qualitätswein* (Q.b.A) which is a quality wine from a named area. Preferably, try to buy *Qualitätswein mit Prädikät* (Q.m.P), which is a natural quality wine with special attributes, made without sugar.

To make your drinking time longer, try mixing an equal amount of white Hock with soda, and adding ice cubes for a long cool drink. White wine mixed with apple juice and chilled is also a most refreshing drink.

There is no data available regarding home-made wines, and it would be very difficult to test these, as they are not made under controlled conditions. As a general rule, I would avoid home-made wines made from roots or leaves, and stick to the fruit- or flower-based wines which produce white wine. For instance, I would avoid elderberry wine, which produces a strong red wine somewhat reminiscent of port, but I would venture to try an elderflower wine, which is light and white.

I have no scientific information regarding cider and perry, but as long as you remember that both these drinks have an alcoholic content, and provided you go for the dry ciders and perries, I think they should present no problem if drunk in moderation.

Cocktails
I think the easiest thing to do with cocktails is to list the most common with their usual ingredients, and mark with a star the ones that should be avoided.

Gin and It	Gin and Italian or French vermouth
Gin Fizz*	Gin and fresh lemon juice
Gimlet	Half dry gin, half lime juice cordial
Campari Soda	Campari, soda water, twist of lemon
Bloody Mary	Vodka and tomato juice with Worcester sauce
Bacardi Cocktail*	2 parts Bacardi rum, 1 part fresh lime juice, 1 part grenadine
Negroni	2 parts gin, 1 part sweet vermouth, 1 part campari with twist of orange
Champagne Cocktail*	Champagne with $\frac{1}{2}$ fl. oz (15 ml) brandy, 1 lump sugar and dash angostura bitters
Bucks Fizz*	Champagne with fresh orange juice

67

Pink Gin	1 part gin, 2 parts water, dash angostura bitters
John Collins*	1 part fresh lemon juice, 3 parts gin, 1 teaspoon castor sugar
Brandy Sour*	1 part lemon juice, 3 parts brandy, ½ teaspoon castor sugar
Whisky Sour*	1 part lemon juice, 3 parts whisky, ½ teaspoon castor sugar, dash angostura bitters
Iceberg	2 parts vodka plus dash of pernod
Manhattan*	1 part dry vermouth, 1 part sweet vermouth, 2 parts Bourbon whisky, dash angostura bitters
Screwdriver*	2 parts vodka, 1 part orange juice
Stinger*	1 part white crème de menthe, 2 parts brandy
Whiskymac*	Half Scotch whisky and half ginger wine
White Lady*	2 parts gin, 1 part lemon juice, 1 part Cointreau, teaspoon egg white
Grenadier*	1 part brandy, 1 part ginger wine
Black Velvet	Half champagne, half Guinness
Martini (American)*	Large measure of gin, dash of dry vermouth, cherry
Martini (English)	Measure of dry vermouth, dash of gin, cherry (can also be served with soda water)

Beers, Lager, Stouts
Beers and lagers do contain vaso-active amines but in

relatively small amounts. The tyramine content has been found to be 2 to 4 mg per litre; as 10 mg tyramine will induce a migraine attack, you would have to drink at least $2\frac{1}{2}$ litres ($4\frac{1}{2}$ pints) of beer to precipitate an attack. However, there are other amines in beers and the cumulative effect of all the amines plus the alcohol content itself could tip the balance on a much lower consumption. So I would say you are fairly safe with beers and lagers, but watch out they don't catch you unawares. I known one lady who enjoyed a regular pint or two and suffered no ill effects at all except during the pre-menstrual period, when half a pint would precipitate an unpleasant migraine attack. Shandy is a good drink for migraine sufferers, especially as the lemonade doesn't contain any real lemon!

Is Guinness good for you? And what of real ale? Unfortunately I could find no data to indicate whether they are better for you or not. I suggest that if you enjoy them, you should drink them until your Attack Form proves otherwise!

8

Other Offenders

YOU HAVE carefully excluded the four main precipitants of migraine: cheese, chocolate, citrus fruits and
alcohol. You are on a high protein diet, and are eating
regular meals/snacks every 3 to 5 hours, thereby eliminating the possibility of low blood sugar, but you are
still getting the occasional unexplained migraine.

There are other foods which contain tyramine,
phenylethylamine and other vaso-active amines which I
have not mentioned in previous chapters because they
are foods which you may only eat occasionally. There are
also a number of foods which we know cause allergic
reactions (not only migraine attacks, but rashes,
nausea, vomiting, or stomach-aches) in many people
who do not necessarily suffer from migraine. We are not
sure what the substance in these foods is that causes
the allergic reaction, but we do know that in a migraine-
sufferer such a reaction can take the form of a full
blown migraine attack.

There are also foods which under normal
circumstances have insignificant levels of vaso-active
amines; but occasionally – perhaps due to growing or
storing conditions – the levels may become unusually
high and can result in an allergic reaction in a
migraine-sufferer. Whenever a sufferer has complained
of an acute reaction to a food which would not normally

be high in these amines, and it has been possible to analyse the offending food, the latter has always been found to have unusually high vaso-active amine levels.

After cheese, chocolate, citrus fruits and alcohol, the next most likely culprit in precipitating a migraine attack is pork. In fact, some migraine-sufferers have found that pork is the only food they cannot tolerate. Pork, of course, includes all pork products: ham, bacon, sausages (even those marked 'beef' often also contain pork – so read the labels carefully), *pâté*, pastes and liver sausage which contain pork meat, fat or liver, frankfurters, hotdogs, pork-based salamis and Continental sausages, cold meats and meat loaves. Pork or ham is used to flavour so many dishes that all labels should be scrutinised to see if the product contains pork. Pea and bean soups often include ham pieces, as do many chicken and turkey pies. Most terrines and *pâtés*, even if they do not include pork meat or liver, are wrapped in bacon.

It is worth remembering that the longer a product has taken to mature the higher the vaso-active amine content is likely to be.

Some sufferers may find they have to avoid pork and pork products altogether; others, like myself, may be able to tolerate small amounts. But beware of the cumulative effects and try not to have pork or ham three meals running, or several days in succession. Give your body a chance to metabolise the difficult food before giving it another dose to deal with!

The following foods are relatively high in the offending amines, but it is not likely they will occur regularly in your daily diet and therefore your reaction to them may not be immediately apparent.

10 mg tyramine is normally required to induce migraine, though it can be very much less. 1 g = 0.0353 oz.

Raspberries

Very high in tyramine. They have 15 to 20 parts per million. About 8 oz are normally enough to precipitate an attack.

Avocado Pears

Tyramine content is 23 mcg per gramme, but they also contain other vaso-active amines: serotonin 10 mcg per gramme and dopamine 4 to 5 mcg per gramme. An average avocado pear would weigh 9 oz (250 g). Normally only half is eaten at a time but this could still account for a substantial intake of vaso-active amines.

Yeast Extracts e.g. Marmite

Yeast itself does not contain tyramine, but the preparation of yeast extract by autolysis and the subsequent fermentation leads to tyramine formation. Marmite contains 1.5 mg per gramme tyramine and 2 mg per gramme histamine which is as high as some cheeses. Also don't forget amines are absorbed better in fat, so bread and butter and Marmite would be more easily absorbed than bread and Marmite on its own.

Pickled Herring

The presence of tyramine in this food can be as high as 3 mg per gramme.

Often the skin or peel of a fruit or vegetable is exceptionally high in amines, while the pulp or flesh has relatively insignificant levels. We have already mentioned this with regard to oranges in Chapter 6 and I now want to draw your attention to others where eating the skin or peel could be hazardous, though you are less likely to get a reaction from eating the flesh alone.

Bananas

Stewed green whole bananas including skins, or over-ripe

bananas baked in their skins, should be avoided. The level of tyramine increases as bananas ripen and is very high in over-ripe ones. Banana skin contains 65 mcg per gramme tyramine plus 50 to 150 mcg per gramme serotonin and 700 mcg per gramme dopamine. The pulp or flesh, in comparison, contains only 7 mcg per gramme tyramine, 28 mcg per gramme serotonin and 8 mcg per gramme dopamine. Migraine-sufferers should thus eat only fresh or medium-ripe bananas without skins.

Broad Beans
Normally, these only produce a reaction when the pod, which contains dopamine, is eaten at the same time.

The following list includes food which contains vaso-active amines, but not normally at significant levels. However, sufferers have reported reactions to these foods in some instances so I list them in case you should also react to them.

Tomatoes
Usually only when you are consuming a large amount of concentrated purée or juice.

Onions
Especially when fried, but also when eaten raw in salads or as a garnish. On the other hand, onions can be rendered harmless if they are blanched before they are eaten. This is done by putting them into cold water, bringing them quickly to the boil, then throwing away the water and using the onions as usual.

Horlicks
Contains similar amounts of tyramine to that contained in oranges and onions.

Red Plums

73

Aubergine/Egg Plant

Monosodium Glutamate
Used for flavouring in many convenience foods and in Chinese dishes.

White Sugar
I personally found a great reduction in the frequency of my attacks when I switched from white sugar to honey for sweetening.

Coffee
I have already discussed the effect of caffeine on low blood sugar in Chapter 3. However, it is amazing how many migraine-sufferers drink large quantities of strong 'real' coffee every day. I recommend changing to a decaffeinated variety if possible, or a 'mild' instant variety. However, some people cannot drink instant coffee at all. This is usually because powdered barley is added to all instant coffees, including the decaffeinated variety. It is the barley which is causing the problem rather than the coffee.

Shellfish
Prawns, shrimps, crab, lobster, mussels, cockles, clams and oysters should all be eaten with care, for many people are allergic to some or all of them.

Gluten
There are a few people who have problems with the gluten in flour. These sufferers tend to have their headaches at absolutely regular intervals every 10 to 12 days, without exception, holiday, no holiday, Sundays or weekdays. Such people often have a history of food fads and problems in childhood, which gradually develop into migraine attacks in adult life.

Some migraine-sufferers say that they react to milk, cream and butter, but there is no real evidence to show why this should be so. I venture to suggest that the cause of the attack might be caused by low blood sugar rather than the food consumed.

I cannot emphasize enough that migraine is almost always caused by a culmination of triggers, and an accumulation of amines in the system which are not metabolised so that, when they reach a critical level, their vaso-activity precipitates a migraine attack.

9

Hormones and Migraine

THIS IS a chapter primarily for women. While it seems unlikely that hormone changes alone can precipitate migraine, they definitely can affect the body's tolerance to specific foods. It may be that you can happily eat all foods throughout the month with the exception of 4 or 5 specific days.

Research[*] has shown that female migraine sufferers (whether or not they have pronounced menstrually-related migraine) have similar hormone levels, and these levels are different from those found in women who do not suffer from migraine.

Migraine sufferers were found to have significantly higher levels of mean plasma oestrogen throughout most of their menstrual cycle, but particularly low levels of progesterone in the late luteal phase when there should normally be a high level. Some studies have found that their levels of mean plasma prolactin, however, were lower than normal throughout the cycle. Experimentally it has been found that ovarian steroids influence prolactin release and the hypothalamic serotoninergic and dopaminergic mechanisms are also involved. Further

[*]Epstein, M. T., Hockaday, J. M., Hockaday, T. D. R., Radcliffe Infirmary, Oxford, 'Migraine and Reproductive Hormones Throughout the Menstrual Cycle', *The Lancet*, 8 March 1975.

research may be able to link these hormonal differences to abnormality in the hypothalamic neurotransmitter mechanisms. This is of special interest as we know that migraine sufferers have difficulty metabolising serotonin and other amines.

While some women suffer only from menstrually-related migraine and so know exactly which days they will have attacks, many women suffer from migraine at other times as well, but are still particularly prone to attacks at certain times in the menstrual cycle.

The changing levels of menstrual hormones appear to be a significant sensitising factor. It is interesting to discover that women taking the oestrogen/progestogen contraceptive pill are particularly sensitive to cheese (48%) and alcohol (28%) precipitating attacks. The incidence of migraine on Day 14 is especially high in this group also. Women who have had a hysterectomy, on the other hand, tend to be more sensitive to fasting (91%) and eating chocolate (47%) before an attack. See Table 5 (and footnote on page 80).

Women who suffer from menstrually-related migraine tend to be those who also suffer from the premenstrual syndrome, with symptoms such as tension, fluid retention (and associated weight gain), breast discomfort and swollen ankles, etc. In fact, it is unusual to have menstrually-related migraine without these other symptoms.

The migraine attacks of these women probably commence with the onset of menstruation and they can expect relief from attacks during middle and late pregnancy. Research at the Radcliffe Infirmary, Oxford, shows that 80% of women sufferers found their migraine completely disappeared during pregnancy after the second missed menstruation, and 60% found significant relief. Unfortunately, there appears to be no significant permanent change or improvement until the menopause.

TABLE 5
Dietary Factors present in Women under 45 years in relation to the Contraceptive Pill and Hysterectomy

	NUMBER OF ATTACKS	CHOCOLATE	CHEESE	CITRUS FRUITS	ALCOHOL	FASTING
		%	%	%	%	%
Takers	262	35	48	20	28	75
Ex-Takers	344	33	44	16	26	73
Non-Takers	488	41	34	18	23	61
Hysterectomy	55	47	29	25	18	91
Probability		< 2.5%	< 0.1%			< 0.1%

$<$ = less than

TABLE 6
Dietary Factors present in the Menstrual Cycle

DAY OF CYCLE	1–4	5–8	9–12	13–15	17–20	21–24	25–28	TOTAL ATTACKS
Chocolate	28*	11	10	16	12	8	5	326
Cheese	29*	14	9	16	11	7	14	349
Citrus Fruits	30*	13	10	11	11	7	17	169
Alcohol	27*	14	9	14	11	7	18	249
Fasting	31*	14	10	12	10	9	14	596

* = Probability exceeds 0.1%

[Tables 5 and 6 taken from *Study of 2313 Spontaneous Migraine Attacks*, Dr Katharina Dalton, February 1975.]

It would seem that pregnancy is the time to indulge oneself in all those delicious chocolates, French cheeses, oranges and grapefruit.

The worst days of the month for migraine attacks are Days 1 to 4 of the menstrual cycle, when 29% of all attacks occur. (Expected incidence if attacks were evenly distributed throughout the cycle would be 14%.) There is a significant increase in sensitivity to all dietary factors in attacks at this time: 31% affected by fasting; 30% by citrus fruit; 29% by cheese; 28% by chocolate; and 27% by alcohol. See Table 6.*

Other possibly sensitive days, of less significance but still worth watching, are those in mid-cycle (when ovulation occurs) and the days immediately preceding and following the period.

As everyone is different, every menstrual cycle is also slightly different. The women whose period lasts eight days will have hormone changes at slightly different times in the cycle from the woman whose period lasts only four days.

While the final precipitating factor triggering a migraine attack is fasting or ingestion of specific food, there are obviously many sensitising factors which may be present at an earlier stage. For example, stress causes alteration in adrenal hormone levels, and lack of sleep or alteration of the diurnal rhythm affects the hypothalamus, which in turn can affect ovarian hormones.

Many women find that they first experience severe migraine when they go on the oestrogen/progestogen contraceptive pill. There are many reasons why this should be, but it is obviously related to an upset in hormonal balance.

*Study of 2313 Spontaneous Migraine Attacks, Dr Katharina Dalton, February 1975.

We know that women with a shortage of progesterone are those most likely to develop menstrually-related migraine. However, it is unfortunate that the man-made progestogen contained in the Pill is *not* the same as the pure progesterone produced by the ovaries (which is not assimilable by mouth). Progestogen is a synthetic substitute which actually lowers the blood progesterone levels, and so makes matters worse. So changing pills to different oesterogen/progestogen combinations will not help at all, and these women would be well advised to try some other means of contraception.

However, without getting drawn too much into the complexities of the Pill, it may be possible to avoid Pill-induced migraines simply by eliminating the foods that I have listed in previous chapters and avoiding low blood sugar situations.

10

General Self-help

Get Yourself Right

THERE is nothing so debilitating as severe pain, and anyone who suffers from migraine will tell you of the utter physical and mental exhaustion that follows a severe migraine attack. Obviously, the body has had a lot to cope with and anyone suffering frequent attacks is bound to find his or her general health is affected.

The body is using all its reserves to cope with attacks, so there may be a sort of general fatigue at other times. Luckily, the body has marvellous recuperative powers if only we give it the right treatment – and that, of course, means attention to diet, coupled with a calm mind.

A few simple changes can make an enormous difference. Try to eat only 100% wholewheat bread. It may taste a little strong to begin with, but you acquire the taste and I'm sure after a few weeks you will not want to eat processed white bread. You will also find it is more filling and satisfying than its white counterpart so that one or two slices will be all you want to eat at one time. However, the phyton contained in wholewheat bread prevents absorption of calcium so you must make certain that calcium deficiency does not result from this change – particularly if you have already been advised to stop eating cheese and milk. Make sure your diet includes plenty of fresh fruit and vegetables and that some of the vegetables are eaten raw in the form of salad every day. Vegetables are most delicious and nutritious when cooked lightly and quickly. We can learn a lot from the Chinese about how to cook vegetables to retain all their crunchiness and goodness.

Regular meals are particularly important for migraine-sufferers – little and often is the rule. In fact many doctors and nutritionists believe that this is best for everyone! Reduce your alcohol consumption – water down drinks with soda, tonic, ginger ale, lemonade, etc. – and always try to drink on a full stomach and not before 6 p.m. Go easy on coffee, too (real and instant), and try to drink decaffeinated instead.

When under stress or overwrought, take a small spoonful of honey to help you raise your blood sugar enough to digest whatever food you eat. Some people also find a couple of spoonfuls of cider vinegar mixed with a little water is a great help to a nervous digestion.

I have found it very beneficial to cut out white sugar. If you have a very sweet tooth, you may throw up your arms in horror at this suggestion, but in fact it is not so difficult. Try using honey for sweetening – it is, in fact, much sweeter than sugar, so you will need to use less and once you have become used to its flavour you will find it is very pleasant in tea and coffee and fruit puddings, pies and cakes.

Once you have established yourself on a healthy, nutritious diet, make sure you incorporate some exercise in your daily life – nothing violent, at least not to start with, and remember the effect exercise has on metabolism and blood sugar. So the rule is gentle exercise, walking, jogging, dancing or swimming and Yoga.

Yoga can have many benefits. It is a very gentle form of exercise where the individual can gradually build up his or her strength and increase the amount of exercise as and when able to do so without straining the body. It is particularly good for those people who have not taken any exercise for a few years. Do not be put off by those complicated postures; you are not expected to be able to do them straight away, and many people who have practised Yoga for years will not be able to do them. That does not mean they are not deriving enormous benefits from the exercises and postures they *can* achieve. The second and almost more important benefit of Yoga is that it teaches relaxation – a condition most migraine-sufferers find hard to achieve, and yet it is especially good for them.

Howard Kent of Yoga for Health Clubs, 9 Old Bond Street, London W1, believes that a lot of the suffering of migraine can be relieved by a controlled programme using Yoga techniques. I am sure that anyone who cares to take up Yoga will find it extremely beneficial and helpful not only for their migraine but for their general health and well-being.

There are also an increasing number of Relaxation for Living classes being held up and down the country. Relaxation cassettes can also be purchased to enable people to learn to relax at home.

What you can do to help yourself in an attack of migraine

The earlier in an attack that you take action, the more likely you are to be able to reduce the pain and length of the attack. First and foremost, try not to panic and become tense in anticipation of the agony you are sure will follow. If you have medication from the doctor, take it immediately; if not, half a teaspoon of table salt plus half a teaspoonful of bicarbonate of soda mixed in a little water often brings some relief. No one knows the reason for this, although bicarbonate of soda is useful in reducing other allergic reactions. A spoonful of honey in a little warm water will not only take away the unpleasant taste of the bicarbonate but will also raise your blood sugar and should help with the nausea and vomiting.

Go to a quiet room, draw the curtains and subdue all light. Try to do the following Yoga head-rolling exercise, which will reduce tension in the neck and shoulders, and increase the flow of blood and oxygen to the brain.

1 Sit down with the back straight.
2 Drop your chin forwards in towards your neck.
3 Now slowly rotate the head in a clockwise direction, making sure that you are not moving your shoulders or the rest of your body.
4 The slower you do this exercise the better it is. If you feel the desire to yawn or sigh – do so. This is a normal and healthy reaction to this exercise.
5 When you have rotated the head in a clockwise direction six times, change and rotate it in an anti-clockwise direction.
6 It is most important that the head be rotated in one direction and then the other.
7 The number of times you do this can be reduced or increased as long as the number is even in each direction.

If you can find a kindly soul to massage your head, scalp, neck and shoulders, this is the best relief you can obtain. I have found it works better than medication. But do not expect results immediately; a quick five-minute massage is no good at all. This must be a slow and gradual massage: first the shoulders and neck to relax them; then systematically all over the scalp. You must guide the person massaging to the painful points so that he or she

85

can work on them in slow, gentle, circular, outward movements dispersing the pressure and tensions. It may be painful at first, but as the pressure points are relieved and the blood flows more freely, so the pain and nausea will subside.

Always rest after an attack to give the body time to recover.

11

Eating Out

THE FIRST thing to remember when eating out, whether it be in a restaurant or with friends, is that you are likely to eat at a different time from your usual meal-time. Even when you have booked a table at a restaurant for 8 p.m. (or your usual dining hour), you will probably find that by the time you have ordered and drunk aperitifs, looked at the menu and ordered your meal, it is 8.30 to 8.45 or even 9 o'clock before you actually *eat* anything. This time factor can be of crucial importance to a migraine-sufferer and I suggest that unless you can be absolutely sure you are going to eat early in the evening (for example, when having dinner before going to the cinema or theatre), you should always have a high protein snack before going out.

Also remember that if you do eat early in the evening before going on to another engagement, you will need to take another snack in the evening (approximately 4 hours after the meal) before retiring. If you forget to do this, you could well wake up the next morning with a migraine due to a plummeting of your blood sugar levels after the evening's activities and a fast of perhaps 13 or 14 hours.

When accepting invitations to dinner-parties, do let your hostess know of your food allergies in advance. For formal occasions when there is a set meal and you cannot find out the menu in advance, take some high protein food, such as a small carton of cottage cheese, with you to eat in the cloakroom if you have had to refuse the main part of the meal. Remember, if you are going to dance the night away or do anything energetic, you will need extra snacks.

When eating out, steer clear of pub lunches unless you know the menu, because so many charming pubs and inns have only a 'ploughman's lunch' (a selection of, usually, hard cheese) or ham or cheese sandwiches. It can be embarrassing not to be able to eat anything that is on offer.

Most 'bought' sandwiches will not contain enough protein for the migraine-sufferer and this is why many say they must have a hot lunch. Good choices for eating out at lunch-time economically are beefburgers (but only those containing 100% minced beef), egg dishes such as omelettes or scrambled eggs, and cottage cheese salad. Turkey contains more protein than chicken, so a turkey sandwich might be suitable.

If you are eating in a restaurant you will have to choose your dishes carefully. Anything in a white sauce is suspect, so always ask the waiter to find out if the sauce contains cheese. Many beef dishes, such as *Boeuf Bourguignon*, will have been made with red wine. Anything cooked with sherry should be avoided, as the heating of wines and sherries seems to increase the amounts of vaso-active amines in them.

Avoid all *gratinée* dishes, French onion soup, which is usually served with toasted cheese as a topping, and minestrone soup, which will probably contain some Parmesan cheese or have it sprinkled on top. When ordering *any* Italian pasta dishes – spaghetti, cannelloni, lasagne – always ask if they contain cheese and ask the waiter not to sprinkle Parmesan cheese on them. Pizzas are not for migraine-sufferers and a lot of people will not be able to tolerate salamis, garlic sausages, etc. Most *pâtés* contain pork meat, fat or bacon, so must also be avoided. Do not order frankfurters and hotdogs, ham rolls, bacon and sausages (even beef sausages usually contain some pork!).

Many Chinese dishes contain monosodium glutamate. If this precipitates an attack for you, then it is best to avoid eating in Chinese restaurants – unless you choose something like Crispy Duck.

If you are having a special meal in a restaurant, you may be tempted to have foods that you would not normally include in your everyday diet – so look out for the special foods listed in Chapter 9 which contain unusually high quantities of vaso-active amines. These include raspberries, bananas cooked in their skins, avocado pears, pickled herrings, aubergines, broad beans, Marmite and other yeast extracts, and shellfish.

Don't risk eating oranges in caramel sauce – the sauce is made with the skins of the oranges, which contain higher levels of amines than the fruit itself. Decline peaches in red wine, pineapple with kirsch, and, of course, chocolate mousses, chocolate profiteroles, chocolate éclairs and gâteaux.

All liqueurs can be a problem to migraine-sufferers, but be especially careful not to have brandy or an orange-based liqueur such as Cointreau or Grand Marnier after your meal.

You can now see how easy it would be to go out for a celebration meal, choosing the following menu:

Avocado vinaigrette

or

Rollmop herrings

or

Pâté

Boeuf Bourguignon
or
Tournedos Rossini
or
Steak Bordelaise

Raspberries and cream
or
Chocolate mousse

Every dish contains migraine precipitant vaso-active amines. You would probably get a very bad attack after a meal like this, but, strangely, would relate the migraine to the excitement and/or stress of going out rather than the meal itself.

All these warnings about foods you must avoid may leave you wondering what foods you can eat, and how you can produce exciting meals for your family, friends and yourself without precipitating a migraine. The recipes and sample menus in the second part of this book will provide a broad variety of delicious dishes, from the plain to the exotic, without triggering a migraine attack.

PART II

Recipes – Defence against Migraine

Recipes:

Defence against Migraine

THE following chapter contains sample menus for breakfasts, lunches, dinners and snacks. By mixing these menus an enormous number of variations for daily eating can be achieved.

Chapters 12 to 15 contain a selection of recipes for breakfasts, main courses, desserts and snacks. However, a recipe in one category might do just as well in another so that you may find that some of the snack menus would make delicious breakfasts, or by increasing the portion would make fine main courses. The choice is up to you. These recipes are just to whet your appetite and show that in spite of dietary restrictions you can still eat delicious meals.

I am listing some of the foods which can be a particular problem to migraine-sufferers, and suggesting ways in which you can modify them or substitute alternatives.

Onions

Many of the recipes contain onions, although there are some migraine-sufferers who find that onions are one of the things that trigger migraine attacks. If you are one of these unlucky people, remember to blanch all onions before using them. This overcomes the problem and you can then proceed with the recipe as directed and suffer no after-effects.

Blanch by peeling the onions, placing them in cold water and bringing to the boil. Throw away the water, drain the onions and use as normal.

Chocolate

Under desserts there are a number of 'chocolate' recipes. These recipes do not, in fact, contain any chocolate but use the admirable substitute, carob powder. Carob tastes very much like chocolate but is much sweeter. Slimmers take note: it has only a little more than half the calories of chocolate and 1% fat as against cocoa's 23.7%. It is composed largely of carbohydrates but contains natural sugars and a generous supply of B vitamins, calcium and other minerals. It has a slightly raw taste similar to that of cocoa powder, but this raw flavour disappears if the powder is mixed with a few drops of cooking oil and a little water, then heated for a few minutes to cook it. Carob powder, sometimes called carob flour, can be obtained from most health food stores but, if in difficulty, contact the Wholefood Shop, Baker Street, London W1, who always have a supply.

If you have a favourite recipe which uses chocolate you may want to adapt it and use carob powder instead. If the recipe originally used cocoa powder, use the same amount of carob powder but reduce the amount of sugar. If the recipe uses sweetened chocolate you will not need to alter the sugar quantity but remember to mix and cook the carob for a few minutes, especially when using in icings, fillings, sauces, etc.

Cheese

In many recipes which call for cheese you can substitute cream or cottage cheese, but the result will tend to be somewhat bland, so you may need to increase the seasoning or include additional herbs and spices.

94

Bananas
Always use bananas which are neither under-ripe nor over-ripe. Do not cook them in their skins or eat the skins, as this is where the highest amounts of amines are concentrated.

Citrus Fruits
If you find that citrus fruits precipitate attacks adapt recipes calling for lemon juice and substitute dry white wine, white wine vinegar or cider vinegar. Lime juice cordial (which contains little if any real lime juice) is another alternative, as is unsweetened apple juice, or lemon juice made from ascorbic acid, not real lemons. Pineapple is a good substitute for grapefruit, and tinned peaches can replace tinned mandarins. Garnish drinks with cherries, fresh peach slices, cucumber or sprigs of mint. Garnish fish dishes with parsley or fennel. Serve duck with black cherries, blackberries or blackcurrants instead of oranges.

For fresh juices, try unsweetened pineapple or apple juice or one of the other non-alcoholic beverages mentioned in Chapter 17.

Brandy
In recipes calling for brandy, try using Tia Maria.

Pork
Veal can be used instead of pork fillet, pork chops or pork joints. For spare ribs use lamb or beef. For pork liver *pâté* substitute a chicken liver *pâté* or a calves' liver *pâté*. In some recipes anchovies can be successfully substituted for bacon or ham.

Sugar
Several recipes specify muscovado sugar, a natural

product available from health food stores and from some supermarkets. White, refined and artificially-coloured sugars should be avoided by migraine-sufferers.

12

Sample Menus

per person

BREAKFASTS

1 glass apple juice
2 scrambled eggs
  Petrovitch (p. 103)
1 slice wholewheat toast
tea/decaffeinated coffee if
  tolerated or milk

---

1 glass vegetable juice
  (V8)
3–4 oz (90–120 g) kidneys
  with mushrooms
  (p. 115)
1 slice wholewheat toast
tea/coffee/milk

---

1 small bowl prunes
2 savoury poached eggs
  (p. 105)
1 slice wholewheat toast
tea/coffee/milk

---

1 fresh pear
1 × 8 oz (240 g) baked
  kipper (p. 113)

1 slice wholewheat bread
  and butter
tea/coffee/milk

---

1 fresh peach
1 × 8 oz (240 g) grilled
  bloater (p. 108)
1 slice wholewheat bread
  and butter
tea/coffee/milk

---

1 glass apple juice
1 × 8 oz (240 g) grilled
  herring (p. 110)
1 slice wholewheat bread
  and butter
tea/coffee/milk

---

1 glass pineapple juice
$3\frac{1}{2}$ oz (105 g) fish capers
  (p. 109)
1 slice wholewheat toast
honey/apricot jam
tea/coffee/milk

1 slice melon
4 oz (120 g) smoked
   haddock
1 slice wholewheat bread
   and butter
tea/coffee/apple juice

-----

1 glass grape juice
2 slices anchovy toast
   (p. 107)
milk

-----

1 glass vegetable juice
   (V8)
1 × 2-egg omelette
   (p. 105)
1 slice wholewheat toast
honey/blackcurrant jam
tea/coffee

-----

1 small bowl dried apricots
2 hard boiled eggs (p. 102)

1 slice wholewheat bread
   and butter
tea/coffee/milk

-----

1 fresh apple
3–4 oz (105–120 g) kidney
   balls (p. 115)
1 slice wholewheat toast
honey/apricot jam
tea/coffee/milk

-----

1 small bunch fresh grapes
4 oz (120 g) herring roe
   fritters (p. 111)
1 slice wholewheat toast
honey/blackberry jam
tea/coffee/milk

-----

1 slice fresh pineapple
4 oz (120 g) kidneys en
   cocotte (p. 116)
1 slice wholewheat toast
tea/coffee/milk

LUNCHES

spaghetti bolognese
   speciale (p. 129)
green salad
small bunch grapes
beverage

-----

stuffed Italian peppers
   (p. 130)
1 baked potato
Wiltshire gooseberry

pudding (p. 167)
beverage

-----

spiced chicken drumsticks
   (p. 148)
green salad
wholewheat bread and
   butter
prune mousse (p. 170)
beverage

-----

salad Niçoise (p. 125)

wholewheat bread and
    butter
almond and apricot lattice
    (p. 153)
____

Polish halibut (p. 121)
mashed potatoes, shredded
    cabbage
blackberry fool (bramble)
    (p. 160)
____

chicken brochettes (p. 140)
mixed salad, rice
blackberry and pear tarts
    (p. 159)
beverage
____

haddock with mushrooms
    (p. 118)
boiled potatoes
pineapple delight (p. 169)
beverage
____

savoury liver (p. 135)
potatoes, peas
gooseberry fool (p. 166)
beverage
____

kidney mince pie (p. 131)
green salad
apricot *kuchen* (p. 157)
beverage

turkey breasts in sour
    cream (p. 151)
potatoes in jacket
endive salad
aromatic fruit salad (p. 159)
beverage
____

Spanish cod steaks (p. 117)
chipped potatoes
watercress and cucumber
    salad
apple tart and cream
____

chicken and mushroom pie
    (p. 139)
mixed vegetables, potato
fresh pineapple slices
____

lamb and apricot kebabs
    (p. 132)
spinach, chips
fresh peach ice cream
    (p. 167)
beverage
____

barbecued spare ribs
    (p. 127)
brown bread
green salad
fresh fruit
beverage

DINNERS

1 slice melon
rosemary lamb casserole
    (p. 134)

peas, baked potato
apricot whip (p. 158)
____

carrot soup
fish pie (p. 125)

99

boiled potatoes, peas or
   salad
fresh peaches or ice cream
   and 'chocolate' sauce
   (p. 174)

---

artichoke hearts salad
roast duck with black
   cherries (p. 137)
beetroot, baked potato in
   jacket
watercress salad
apricot sorbet (p. 157)

---

grape and chicory salad
barbecued beef kebabs
   (p. 126)
rice
apple cheesecake (p. 154)

Italian pepper salad
grilled chicken (p. 144)
new potatoes, broccoli
cherry almond tarts
   (p. 162)

---

celery with cream cheese
spiced turkey (p. 152)
rice, endive or green salad
chestnut pears (p. 168)

---

cauliflower raisin salad
Italian chicken breasts
   (p. 145)
button mushrooms and
   peas
strawberry ice pudding
   (p. 171)

cucumber salad
roast chicken with peaches
   (p. 147)
rice, spinach salad
gooseberry cream (p. 165)

---

watercress soup (p. 200)
shepherds pie (p. 128)
peas, carrots
pineapple custards (p. 168)

---

corn on the cob
Mexican chicken in the
   brick (p. 146)
rice, green salad
blackcurrant ice cream
   (p. 161)

---

cauliflower and almond
   soup (p. 198)
fillet of sole Margaretta
   (p. 124)
sauté potato, spinach
strawberry shortcakes
   (p. 172)

---

leeks with cream cheese
fillet of lamb Dijon
   (p. 132)
peas and potatoes
fresh fruit

---

mushroom salad
chicken with cashew nuts
   (p. 143)
rice
blackcurrant lattice
   (p. 161)

mushroom soup (p. 199)
Wiener schnitzel (p. 136)
chicory and watercress
  salad

French fried potatoes
cherry ginger jelly (p. 163)

SAMPLE SNACKS

Mid-morning

1 cream cheese and walnut
sandwich (p. 197) *or*
1 Scotch egg (p. 188) *or*
1 sweet-sour chicken
drumstick (p. 183) *or*
1 slice kipper quiche
(p. 190) *or*
2 cream cheese and date
scones (p. 181) *or*
2 oz (60 g) cottage delight
(p. 180) *or*
1 bumper decker sandwich
(p. 196)

Mid-afternoon

1 French sardine sandwich
(p. 197) *or*
1 cream cheese sandwich
(p. 196) *or*
1 mushroom cheese on toast
(p. 182) *or*

chicken liver *pâté* on 1 slice
toast (p. 183) *or*
2–3 oz (60–90 g) anchovy
mousse (p. 189) *or*
slice smoked haddock flan
(p. 194) *or*
portion piperade (p. 187)

Late Evening

cream of watercress soup
(p. 200) plus one slice
wholewheat bread *or*
cream of cauliflower and
almond soup (p. 198) plus
one slice wholewheat bread
or
1 poached egg with spinach
(p. 187) *or*
1 beef and mushroom pasty
(p. 177) *or*
2 oz (60 g) herring roes on
toast (p. 190) *or*
1 tartar burger (p. 179) *or*
portion of tuna fish and
sweetcorn flan (p. 195)

101

13

Breakfast Dishes

MANY people cannot face the thought of eating anything for breakfast. It takes a little time to get used to new eating habits, but remember breakfast doesn't have to be an elaborate meal, requiring complicated recipes, but should simply be high in protein. Eggs are ideal for a quick, easy and satisfying breakfast. You will probably need to eat 2 eggs to fulfil your protein requirement; these can be hard or soft boiled, coddled, poached or served in a variety of other ways. Soft boiled eggs will take between $3\frac{1}{2}$ and 4 minutes to cook depending on whether you put them into cold water and bring to the boil, or directly into boiling water. Hard boiled eggs take about 12 minutes and coddled eggs 6 to 8 minutes. So you see a nourishing breakfast can be prepared in a very short time.

EGG DISHES

Scrambled Eggs Petrovitch   *Serves 2*

4 standard eggs   chopped chives (or spring
paprika   onions)
ground black pepper   knob of butter
sea salt   wholewheat toast

Scrambling eggs is quick and easy to do, but you must always cook over a low heat, stir continuously and serve quickly.

Whisk the eggs with a fork or egg-whisk until frothy. Add a pinch of paprika, a pinch of ground black pepper and salt to taste. Chop the chives and keep on one side.

Put a knob of butter into a saucepan (preferably non-stick) and heat until it melts. Add the egg mixture. Cook over a low heat, stirring frequently with a wooden fork or spoon. In about 2 minutes the eggs will become 'shiny' and smooth in texture. Serve at once on to hot buttered wholewheat toast and garnish with the chopped chives.

Cheesy Scrambled Eggs   *Serves 2*

1 oz (30 g) butter   pinch powdered tarragon
4 eggs   salt and paprika

2 oz (60 g) cream cheese
a few drops Worcester
   sauce

2 slices wholewheat toast
chopped parsley, for
   garnish

Melt the butter in a saucepan. Beat the eggs and then add the cream cheese, Worcester sauce, tarragon, salt and paprika. Try to break down the cream cheese as much as possible before adding the egg mixture to the melted butter in the saucepan. Proceed as for ordinary scrambled eggs, stirring the mixture all the time. If necessary add a little milk.

Meanwhile, toast 2 slices of wholewheat bread and butter them. When the egg mixture is firm but still soft and creamy, serve immediately on to the buttered wholewheat toast. Garnish with chopped parsley.

Pimento Eggs   *Serves 2*

$\frac{1}{2}$ small red pimento
$\frac{1}{2}$ green pepper
4 eggs
4 dessertspoons milk
pinch of cayenne pepper
pinch of sea salt

pinch of dry mustard
dash of Tabasco sauce
1 to 2 oz (30 to 60 g)
   butter
1 small onion, finely
   chopped

Chop the red pimento and the green pepper into small pieces, discarding the seeds. Whisk the eggs, add the milk and season with the cayenne pepper, salt and dry mustard. Add a dash of Tabasco sauce.

Put the butter in a frying pan and when melted, add the beaten eggs. Stirring all the time, add the chopped onion and mix well. When the eggs are cooked but still soft and creamy, add the pimento and green pepper pieces. Stir in for only a minute or two, then serve immediately.

Plain Omelette   *Serves 2*

4 eggs
salt and freshly-ground
    black pepper
knob of butter

Break the eggs into a bowl and whisk until frothy; add salt and pepper to taste. Put a knob of butter into a frying pan, using enough to cover the bottom of the pan when melted. Heat until the melted butter begins to smoke. Add the egg mixture quickly and cook over moderate heat, allowing the omelette to set for about $1\frac{1}{2}$ to 2 minutes. As soon as the underside of the omelette is firm, fold the edges into the centre using a spatula or bread knife. Cook for a further 1 to 2 minutes. Serve at once.

Many different omelettes can be easily made by adding sauté vegetables before folding, e.g. mushrooms, potato, onion, chicken pieces, or flaked fish.

Savoury Poached Eggs   *Serves 1*

2 standard eggs
4 anchovies
wholewheat bread

Always use fresh eggs for poaching and preferably not from a cold refrigerator.

Break the eggs into a cup and slip them into a pan of boiling water (some people add a tablespoon of vinegar to the water as this prevents the white of the egg frothing). Simmer very gently for about 3 minutes.

105

Separately grill 4 anchovies on buttered wholewheat toast until hot.

Remove the eggs with a perforated spoon and place on to the hot anchovies.

FISH DISHES

Anchovy Toast *Serves 2*

1 oz (30 g) anchovies   cayenne pepper
1 oz (30 g) butter   slices of wholewheat toast
2 large egg yolks

Pound the anchovies and butter into a smooth paste (this can be done in a blender). Melt the anchovy butter in a small saucepan and as it melts add the beaten-up yolks. Stir until the mixture becomes creamy. Add cayenne pepper to taste and spread thickly on slices of wholewheat toast.

Baked Fish Fillet *Serves 3 to 4*

1 to 1¼ lb (480 to 600 g)   1 to 2 oz (30 to 60 g)
   fish fillet   butter
salt   chopped chives or fennel,
white pepper   for garnish

Wash fresh fillets or thaw frozen fillets and if necessary cut into slices about ¾ in (19 mm) thick. Place the fish fillets in an ovenproof dish. Season with salt and pepper

107

and cover with the butter. Cover the dish with a lid or baking foil. Cook in oven at Gas 6/400°F/200°C for 15 to 20 minutes.

Garnish with chopped chives or fennel.

Bloater Capers   *Serves 2*

1 × 8 to 10 oz (240 to 300 g) bloater or 2 smaller bloaters
1 egg

1 teaspoon capers, chopped
salt and freshly ground pepper

Flake the flesh of the bloater, discarding the bones and skin. Separate the egg and mix the beaten egg yolk with the fish. Season with salt and pepper. Beat the egg white until stiff and fold into the fish mixture. Butter some scallop shells or a shallow ovenproof dish and place the chopped capers at the bottom. Fill up the shells or dish with the fish mixture and bake in a moderately hot oven Gas 5/375°F/190°C for 10 to 15 minutes.

Grilled Bloaters   *Serves 2*

2 bloaters
2 dessertspoons breadcrumbs
$\frac{1}{2}$ teaspoon dry mustard

1 small onion, chopped
$\frac{1}{2}$ teaspoon chopped parsley
4 knobs butter

Cut the heads and tails off the bloaters. Split them open and take out the backbone. Mix the breadcrumbs, mustard, chopped onion and parsley together and sprinkle the mixture on to the bloaters. Put 2 knobs of butter on each bloater and grill them for 10 to 15 minutes.

Cod Scallops *Serves 2*

1½ oz (45 g) butter
7 oz (210 g) cod fillets,
  boned
1 dessertspoon wholewheat
  flour
½ pint (300 ml) milk
½ teaspoon anchovy sauce

1 teaspoon cider vinegar
mustard powder, cayenne
  pepper and black
  pepper
scallop shells
breadcrumbs

Melt the butter in a saucepan. Flake the cod fillets into this together with the flour. Gradually add the milk. Season with the anchovy sauce and cider vinegar. Sprinkle in a little mustard powder, cayenne pepper and freshly ground black pepper. Cook until the mixture is of a thick consistency. Grease some scallop shells. Put the mixture into them and top it with a layer of breadcrumbs. Brown under the grill.

Fish Capers *Serves 1*

4 oz (120 g) cod fillet
  (fresh or frozen)
1 dessertspoon mayonnaise
1 dessertspoon capers

Steam the fish in a little water for 10 minutes. (If preferred, the fish can be grilled.) Put the cooked fish on to a hot plate. Pour on the mayonnaise. Garnish with capers.

Grilled Herrings

Serves 4

4 herrings
1 tablespoon sunflower oil
1 oz (30 g) butter
½ oz (15 g) wholewheat
    flour

½ teaspoon French mustard
¼ pint (150 ml) water
2 tablespoons cider vinegar
salt and freshly ground
    pepper

Clean the herrings and brush with the sunflower oil. Cook the herrings under a hot grill for 7 to 9 minutes until golden brown. Turn over after 4 minutes so that both sides brown.

In the meantime melt the butter in a saucepan, take off the heat, and add the flour and mustard, stirring all the time, gradually add the water and then the vinegar. Season to taste with salt and the freshly ground pepper. Bring to the boil, stirring continuously, and cook for a few minutes. Serve poured over the grilled herrings.

Grilled Marinated Herrings

Serves 2 to 3

2 lb (960 g) herring

Marinade
7 to 10 tablespoons oil
1 tablespoon cider vinegar
1 tablespoon dry white
    wine

1 small onion, sliced
2 teaspoons salt
1 teaspoon ground pepper
slices of buttered
    wholewheat bread

Wash and scale the fresh fish (gut if necessary). Fillet the fish. Do not remove the skin. Score the fillets in 3 or 4 places. Mix the marinade and pour it over the fillets. Leave to marinate for 2 hours. Remove the marinated fish fillets and place under a hot grill skin side nearest the

110

heat. Baste with the marinade. Grill for about 8 minutes. Serve hot with buttered wholewheat bread.

This recipe is also excellent with mackerel, salmon trout, trout, plaice or sole.

Creamy Herring Roes   *Serves 2 to 4*

8 oz (240 g) soft herring   ½ oz (15 g) butter
  roes   ½ oz (15 g) plain flour
¼ pint (150 ml) milk   1 dessertspoon chopped
salt and freshly ground   fresh parsley
  black pepper   hot buttered wholewheat
                               toast

Wash the roes, if using tinned roes, drain them. Put the roes with the milk in a pan and simmer for 5 to 10 minutes. Drain and put the liquid on one side. Wash the roes and season with salt and freshly ground black pepper. Put the butter in a pan and when it has melted, draw from the heat, stir in the flour and gradually add the roe liquid, stirring all the time. Bring to the boil and add the roes and half the parsley. Cook for a few minutes. Serve on slices of hot buttered wholewheat toast and sprinkle chopped parsley over the top.

Herring Roe Fritters   *Serves 2 to 4*

8 oz (240 g) soft or hard   2 oz (60 g) butter
  herring roes   watercress
salt and freshly ground   hot buttered wholewheat
  black pepper   toast
¼ pint (150 ml) coating
  batter

111

Wipe the roes, season with salt and freshly ground black pepper and dip them into the batter. Put the butter in a frying pan, add a little extra cooking oil and when the fat is smoking hot, fry the fritters until golden brown. Serve on slices of buttered wholewheat toast and garnish with sprigs of watercress.

Herrings with Chutney   *Serves 4*

4 herrings   salt and pepper
2 dessertspoons sweet   ½ oz (15 g) butter
  chutney

Clean the herrings, split in half and remove the backbone. Spread the chutney on the inside of each herring. Season with salt and pepper and close up the herrings. Brush each herring with a little melted butter and cook under a hot grill for 7 to 10 minutes, turning once.

(Contributed by Jill F. Middleton.)

Fish Cakes   *Serves 3 to 4*

12 oz (360 g) cooked   salt and pepper
  flaked fish   1 small egg
4 oz (120 g) potato,   breadcrumbs
  mashed   cooking oil
1 oz (30 g) butter   sprigs of parsley and slices
2 teaspoons chopped   of tomato
  parsley

Mix the mashed potato with the flaked fish, discarding all bones and skin. Melt the butter and add it to the fish mixture, add the chopped parsley, season with salt and pepper. Bind the mixture together with a little beaten egg and divide into small flat cakes or croquettes. Coat with egg, then dip them into breadcrumbs. Deep fry in smoking hot fat until golden brown. Drain well and serve with sprigs of parsley and slices of tomato.

Kedgeree   *Serves 2*

2 oz (60 g) butter
1 oz (30 g) plain flour
¾ pint (450 ml) milk
salt and pepper
1 teaspoon anchovy sauce
2 eggs

8 oz (240 g) smoked
    haddock
4 oz (120 g) boiled long
    grain rice
sprigs fresh parsley

Melt the butter in a saucepan, take off the heat and add the flour. Gradually add the milk, stirring all the time. Season well with salt and pepper and anchovy sauce. Bring to the boil and cook briefly.

Meanwhile hard boil the eggs, cut them in half and put the yolks on one side. Chop up the whites and add them to the milk mixture. Poach the fish, then remove skin and bones and flake the flesh. Add it to the milk. Now add the boiled rice and stir for several minutes until everything is hot. Serve with the egg yolks grated over the top and garnish with sprigs of parsley.

Baked Kippers   *Serves 2*

2 × 6 oz (180 g) kippers
1 oz (30 g) butter

slices of buttered
    wholewheat bread

113

Sandwich the kippers in pairs with knobs of butter in between, wrap in cooking foil and bake in a hot oven Gas 7/425°F/220°C for about 15 minutes. Serve at once with slices of buttered wholewheat bread.

Kipper Scramble   *Serves 2*

6 oz (180 g) kipper fillets   salt and freshly ground
1 oz (30 g) butter   black pepper
2 large eggs   hot buttered wholewheat
1 tablespoon milk   toast
chopped parsley

Poach the kipper fillets, drain and put on one side. Melt butter in a pan. Beat the egg and milk together and add the flaked poached fillets, chopped parsley, salt and pepper.

Add the mixture to the butter in the pan and scramble over a low heat for about 5 minutes. Serve on hot buttered wholewheat toast.

MEAT DISHES

Kidney Balls   *Serves 2*

4 oz (120 g) ox kidney   1 large egg
1 leek   oil for frying
salt and freshly ground
    black pepper

Chop the kidney into small pieces. Finely chop the leek
and mix the two together.
    Season with salt and freshly ground black pepper and
bind the whole together with an egg, well beaten. Divide
into balls and fry in hot oil.

Kidneys with Mushrooms   *Serves 2*

7 oz (210 g) ox kidney   salt and pepper
1 oz (30 g) butter   dried mixed herbs
4 oz (120 g) mushrooms   2 slices wholewheat toast
stock cube   parsley

Cut the kidney into small pieces, discarding all the fat.
Roll the pieces in flour. Heat the butter in a saucepan,
add the kidney and fry gently. After a few minutes add

115

the mushrooms (washed and cut into slices). Dissolve a stock cube in a little water and add it to the saucepan to make a rich gravy. Add salt, pepper and herbs to taste. Cook for 10 to 15 minutes, then serve on slices of wholewheat toast garnished with chopped parsley.

Kidneys en Cocotte   *Serves 4*

2 lamb's kidneys
1 oz (30 g) butter
1 tablespoon finely
   chopped fresh chives
4 eggs

1 small carton
   (5 fl.oz/150 ml) sour
   cream
2 tablespoons milk
salt and freshly ground
   black pepper

Skin and cut up the kidneys into small pieces. Put the butter into a frying pan over a high heat. Fry the kidney pieces very quickly to seal them, then remove them from the pan. Divide the pieces into four and put them in 4 ramekin dishes. Cover each with a layer of the chopped chives. Carefully break an egg into each dish on top of the kidneys and chives. Mix the milk and sour cream together and season with salt and pepper. Spoon this mixture over the eggs.

Bake in a medium oven Gas 4/350°F/180°C for about 15 minutes until the eggs are set.

14

Main Courses

Spanish Cod Steaks   *Serves 4*

4 × 4 oz (120 g) cod steaks
2 oz (60 g) butter
1 small onion, finely
  chopped
1 × 8 oz (227 g) can
  tomatoes
2 tablespoons natural
  apple juice

thyme
clove of garlic, crushed
dessertspoon freshly
  chopped parsley
salt and freshly ground
  black pepper
a few gherkins and stuffed
  olives

Fry the cod steaks in butter for about 15 minutes. When cooked, place them in an ovenproof dish and keep hot. Add the rest of the butter to the pan, then add the chopped onion. When it is transparent but not brown, add the tomatoes chopped into small pieces. Add the natural apple juice, a pinch of thyme, the garlic, parsley and salt and pepper. Add as much of the juice from the tinned tomatoes as is necessary to give the sauce a smooth consistency.

When the sauce is cooked, pour it over the fish. Garnish with the gherkins and stuffed olives.

Haddock with Mushrooms

Serves 4

2 lb (960 g) filleted fresh
   haddock
$\frac{1}{4}$ pint (150 ml) water
4 tablespoons dry cider
1 lb (480 g) mushrooms
1 oz (30 g) onion, chopped
   and blanched
1 dessertspoon chopped
   fresh parsley

$2\frac{1}{2}$ oz (75 g) butter
$\frac{1}{2}$ oz (15 g) plain flour
$\frac{1}{2}$ pint (300 ml) hot milk
salt and pepper
1 teaspoon paprika
2 oz (60 g) cream cheese
sprigs of parsley for
   garnish

Divide the fish into 4 portions and place in an ovenproof dish. Pour the $\frac{1}{4}$ pint (150 ml) water and the dry cider over it. Take a few of the mushrooms and slice them over the top. Put a lid on the dish and cook in a hot oven, Gas 8/450°F/230°C for about 15 minutes.

Meanwhile finely chop the rest of the mushrooms, mix them with the onion and chopped parsley. Melt 2 oz (60 g) butter in a saucepan and cook the mushroom mixture gently for 2 or 3 minutes then put on one side.

When the fish is cooked, drain off the liquid and boil it for 7 minutes. Keep the fish hot. Melt $\frac{1}{2}$ oz (15 g) butter in a saucepan. Add the flour and, stirring all the time, gradually add the hot milk and about $\frac{1}{4}$ pint (150 ml) of the reduced fish liquid. Simmer for about 5 minutes. Season to taste with salt and pepper, then add the paprika. Add the cream cheese. Stir until a smooth consistency is acquired.

Stir about half of the sauce into the mushroom mixture and pour it into the bottom of a serving dish. Place the fish on top and pour over the remainder of the sauce. Garnish with paprika sprinkled over and sprigs of parsley. Serve with boiled potatoes.

Indian Curried Haddock   *Serves 4*

1 clove garlic
3 oz (90 g) onion, chopped
1 tablespoon melted
  butter/cooking oil
2 tablespoons curry
  powder
salt and pepper

1 oz (30 g) plain flour
4 fillets haddock, fresh or
  smoked
2 tomatoes
slices of cucumber, to
  garnish

Finely chop the garlic then add 1 oz (30 g) chopped onion and the melted butter or cooking oil and mix with the curry powder to make a paste. Add salt and pepper to taste. Rub this paste over the fish fillets, dust them in flour then fry in hot fat for 8 to 10 minutes until cooked.

Wash the tomatoes and chop into small pieces. Mix with the rest of the chopped onion and season with salt and pepper. Serve this mixture cold with the hot fish and garnish with slices of cucumber.

(Contributed by Jill F. Middleton.)

Parisian Fish Salad   *Serves 6*

1 lb (480 g) fresh haddock,
  cooked
1 onion, finely chopped
4 oz (120 g) new potatoes,
  cooked and diced
2 gherkins, finely chopped

¼ pint (150 ml) mayonnaise
1 lettuce
1 hard boiled egg
2 tomatoes, chopped
green olives, capers and
  fresh parsley

Flake the fish and blend with the onion, potatoes and gherkins. Add half the mayonnaise and mix well. Wash the lettuce and arrange in a salad bowl. Place the fish

119

mixture in the centre of the lettuce. Pour more mayonnaise over and decorate with slices of hard boiled egg, tomato, green olives, capers and parsley.

Brittany Halibut
Serves 6

2 oz (60 g) butter
2 oz (60 g) onion, chopped
1 oz (30 g) flour
1 wineglass dry white wine
2 cloves garlic
2 tablespoons chopped
  fresh parsley

salt
cayenne pepper
2 lb (960 g) halibut,
  filleted
$\frac{1}{4}$ pint (150 ml) cooking oil
$\frac{1}{2}$ lb (240 g) small tomatoes

Melt the butter in a saucepan and cook the chopped onion in it until it is soft but not brown. Stir in the flour and gradually add the wine, stirring all the time. Simmer for 5 minutes, then add the garlic and parsley. Season with salt and cayenne pepper. Add a little more wine if necessary. Flour the fish lightly and fry in hot cooking oil until golden (about 3 minutes on each side). Place on a shallow ovenproof dish and cover with the sauce. Make an edging with tomato wedges. Bake in a preheated hot oven Gas 7/425°F/220°C, for a few minutes. Serve sprinkled with freshly chopped parsley.

(Contributed by Jill F. Middleton.)

Polish Halibut *Serves 4*

1½ lb (720 g) filleted
  halibut steaks
4 oz (120 g) horseradish,
  grated
¼ oz (7 g) butter
¼ oz (7 g) flour
¼ pint (150 ml) hot milk
¼ pint (150 ml) cream

3 raw egg yolks
salt and freshly ground
  black pepper
1 tablespoon natural apple
  juice
1 hard boiled egg yolk,
  chopped
chopped fresh parsley

Divide the fish into 4 steaks and put in a pan. Cover with water and poach for about 10 minutes until cooked. Drain the liquid and boil until it is reduced by one-third. Keep the fish hot. Add the horseradish to the liquor and simmer for 10 minutes. In another pan, melt the butter, remove from the flame and stir in the flour. Gradually add the hot milk, stirring all the time. Return to the flame. When the sauce is smooth and cooked, add the horseradish sauce, the cream and the raw egg yolks and season with salt and pepper. Keep over a low heat, stirring continuously for a few more minutes, then remove from the heat and add the natural apple juice. The sauce should be very creamy. Coat the fish with the sauce and garnish with the chopped hard boiled egg yolk and parsley sprinkled over. Served with mashed potatoes and shredded cabbage.

(Contributed by Jill F. Middleton.)

Poached Salmon Steaks with Cucumber Sauce   *Serves 4*

2 oz (60 g) butter
1 small onion, finely
    chopped
1 medium carrot, chopped
2 pints (1.2 l) water
½ pint (300 ml) dry white
    wine
1 level teaspoon salt
6 white peppercorns
4 × 4 oz (120 g) salmon
    steaks
cress

For the sauce
1 teaspoon onion, finely
    chopped
2 tablespoons white wine
    vinegar
½ teaspoon salt
¼ teaspoon Tabasco
¼ pint (150 ml)
    ready-whipped cream
1 cucumber

Melt the butter in a saucepan. Add the vegetables and
cook slowly for 5 minutes without browning. Add the
water, wine, salt and peppercorns. Simmer for another 5
minutes. Put the salmon steaks into the pan and simmer
very slowly for about 20 minutes, then lift out carefully
and drain. Allow to get quite cold and then remove the
skin.

For the sauce: Mix the onion with the vinegar, salt and
Tabasco. Fold lightly into the cream. Peel and grate the
cucumber. Drain thoroughly and then fold into the sauce.
Chill.

To serve: pour or spoon the sauce over the salmon steaks
and garnish with cress.

(Contributed by Jill F. Middleton.)

Salmon Salad   *Serves 4*

2 × 7½ oz (212 g) cans of
  salmon
½ small red pepper,
  chopped
2 tablespoons mango
  chutney
2 oz (60 g) stuffed cocktail
  olives
bunch of watercress
¼ pint (150 ml) sour cream
2 tablespoons wine vinegar
1 dessertspoon chopped
  fresh chives
salt and freshly ground
  black pepper

Drain the liquid from the salmon and flake the flesh up
in a bowl. Add the red pepper, chutney and stuffed
olives. Mix together well. Line a serving plate with the
watercress and pile the salmon mixture in the centre.

Make a dressing for the salmon by blending together
the sour cream, vinegar and chives. Season with salt and
freshly ground black pepper. The dressing can either be
spooned over the salmon or handed in a dish separately.

N.B. Tuna fish can be substituted for the salmon to
make a more economical dish.

Salmon Soufflé   *Serves 4*

1 lb (480 g) potatoes
1 × 8 oz (227 g) can of red
  salmon
2 large eggs
1 oz (30 g) butter
1 tablespoon freshly
  chopped parsley
salt and freshly ground
  black pepper

Boil the potatoes. Mash the salmon. Separate the eggs,
add the yolks to the salmon, keeping the whites on one
side. Mash the butter and potatoes, then add the salmon

mixture and parsley. Season with salt and pepper. Beat the egg whites until stiff, then fold into the salmon mixture. Place in a soufflé dish and bake in the oven Gas 5/375°F/190°C for 30 to 35 minutes. Serve with a green salad.

Fillet of Sole Margaretta *Serves 4*

¼ pint (150 g) sunflower oil
4 large fillets of sole
salt and pepper
4 oz (120 g) mushrooms, finely chopped
1 shallot or small onion, finely chopped

1 oz (30 g) butter
2 oz (60 g) canned sweet corn
paprika
fresh chopped parsley

Put the oil in a pan and heat. Season the fillets with salt and pepper, and fry gently in the oil until cooked (about 3 minutes each side). Drain well, place on a serving dish and keep warm. Wash and finely chop the mushrooms and add them to the chopped shallot/onion. Gently cook this mixture in the butter until tender, but do not brown. Stir in the tinned sweet corn and season with salt and pepper.

Pour the sauce over the fish, sprinkle with paprika and decorate with fresh chopped parsley.

(Contributed by Jill F. Middleton.)

Salad Niçoise

Serves 2 to 4

1 lettuce
7½ oz (212 g) can of tuna
   fish
2 hard boiled eggs
10 black olives
6 anchovy fillets
½ red pepper, chopped
8 radishes, cut in rosettes
a few capers
a small piece of chopped
   fennel
chopped chives

For the dressing
clove of garlic
wine vinegar
olive oil
salt and freshly ground
   black pepper
¼ teaspoon clear honey

Wash the lettuce and cut into quarters. Arrange in the salad bowl. Drain the tuna fish and divide into pieces, add it to the lettuce together with slices of hard boiled egg. Add the rest of the ingredients to make a decorative salad.

Make up a French dressing with the above ingredients and toss the salad in it just before serving.

Fish Pie

Serves 4

1 oz (30 g) butter
3 shallots or small onions,
   finely chopped
¼ pint (150 ml) white wine
   (Chablis or Graves)
1½ lb (720 g) mixed white
   fish, skinned and boned
6 oz (180 g) puff pastry

For the sauce
1 oz (30 g) butter
1 oz (30 g) flour
fish liquid
¼ pint (150 ml) single
   cream
salt and freshly ground
   pepper

Heat 1 oz (30 g) butter in a saucepan and fry the chopped shallots. Add the wine. Break the mixed fish into pieces and add to the mixture. Cook for about 5 minutes. Lift fish out of the liquid and put into a 2-pint pie dish.

For the sauce, melt 1 oz (30 g) butter, remove from heat, and stir in the flour. Gradually add the fish liquid and cream. Season with salt and freshly ground pepper. Cook slowly until thickened, stirring continuously. Pour over the fish. Cover the pie with the puff pastry and bake for 20 minutes at Gas 6/400°F/200°C, then another 10 to 15 minutes at Gas 5/375°F/190°C.

(Contributed by Jill F. Middleton.)

Barbecued Beef Kebabs *Serves 2*

9 oz (270 g) fillet or rump steak
salt and freshly ground black pepper
Worcester sauce
cooking oil

For the sauce
2 dessertspoons cooking oil
2 small cloves garlic, finely chopped
2 dessertspoons ground ginger
1 dessertspoon ground cumin seed
2½ teaspoons honey
1 dessertspoon ground rice
2 tablespoons wine vinegar
1 dessertspoon tomato paste
1 teaspoon soy sauce
water to thin as necessary
1 teaspoon dessicated coconut

Cut the fillet or rump steak into squares and place on 2 skewers. Sprinkle with salt, freshly ground black pepper and a few drops of Worcester sauce and dribble over a few drops of cooking oil. Cook under a hot grill for about 10 to 15 minutes, turning once or twice so that the meat is cooked on both sides.

Meanwhile, heat 2 dessertspoons cooking oil in a pan with the finely chopped garlic. Do not brown. Add the ground ginger, cumin seed and honey. Mix thoroughly and add the ground rice. Stirring all the time, add the vinegar, tomato paste and soy sauce. Simmer gently and thin with water if necessary. Add the dessicated coconut and continue to cook gently for an hour. Do not allow to burn.

Pour the sauce over the cooked kebabs and serve on a bed of rice or with pieces of fresh bread and a green salad.

Barbecued Spare Ribs

Serves 4

2 tablespoons sunflower oil
6 oz (180 g) onion, finely chopped
1 beef stock cube
3 tablespoons clear honey
$\frac{1}{4}$ pint (150 ml) hot water
1 crushed clove garlic

4 teaspoons chilli powder
$\frac{1}{4}$ teaspoon ground ginger
2 tablespoons tomato paste
vinegar
2 lb (960 g) spare ribs
(lamb or beef)

Put the oil in a saucepan and add the onion. Cook gently until tender but do not brown. Meanwhile dissolve the stock cube and honey in the hot water. Add the garlic, chilli powder and ginger to the onions. Stirring all the time, add the tomato paste, the vinegar and the stock cube mix. Simmer gently for about 10 minutes.

Put the spare ribs in one layer in a roasting tin and spoon a little of the sauce over them. Roast in a medium hot oven Gas 5/375°F/190°C for 30 minutes. Pour off the excess fat and spoon the remaining sauce over the ribs. Cook for another hour at the same temperature.

(Contributed by Jill F. Middleton.)

Shepherds Pie *Serves 4*

2 medium onions
8 oz (240 g) mushrooms
2 tablespoons cooking oil
1 lb (480 g) minced beef
1 × 14 oz (397 g) can of
 tomatoes
½ teaspoon mixed herbs

salt and freshly ground
 black pepper
1 Oxo cube
few drops caramel
 colouring
1½ lbs (720 g) potatoes
1½ oz (45 g) butter

Skin and finely chop the onions. Wash the mushrooms and chop them up.

Put the oil in the pan and gently fry the onions without browning them. When they are transparent, add the mince, mushrooms and tomatoes from the tin. Mash the tomatoes into the mixture and gradually add the tomato juice from the tin. Mix with a wooden spoon. Add the herbs, salt and freshly ground black pepper, and crumble the Oxo cube. Cook for 30 to 45 minutes until the mixture is moist but not runny. Add a few drops of colouring.

Meanwhile peel the potatoes and boil them in water. When cooked, add the butter and salt and pepper and mash into a smooth paste.

Put the mince mixture into a pie dish. Cover with the mashed potato and put the pie under the grill for 10 minutes until well browned.

Spaghetti Bolognese Speciale   *Serves 4*

2 tablespoons olive oil
1 large onion, finely
  chopped
1 large clove garlic, finely
  chopped
1 lb (480 g) raw minced
  beef
1 large (14 oz/397 g) can
  tomatoes, peeled
3 oz (90 g) anchovies,
  chopped

1 dessertspoon capers,
  chopped
2 oz (60 g) black olives
1 teaspoon basil
$\frac{1}{2}$ teaspoon honey
salt and freshly ground
  black pepper
1 lb (480 g) spaghetti
4 oz (120 g) carton cottage
  cheese

Heat oil in saucepan and gently fry the onion and finely chopped garlic until yellow and translucent. Add the raw minced beef. Drain the tomatoes and add them to the pan, chopping them into pieces with a fork. Keep the juice on one side.

Add the chopped anchovies, capers, olives, basil and honey. Stir well, add salt and freshly ground pepper and the tomato juice as necessary, but maintaining a fairly thick consistency.

Meanwhile, cook the spaghetti in a large panful of boiling water to which you have added a couple of drops of oil. Do not overcook. It should be just tender but *not* sticky. This faint 'bite' is what the Italians call *al dente*.

Serve on plates with the spaghetti making a nest for the sauce and topped with two teaspoons of cottage cheese.

Stuffed Italian Peppers   *Serves 2*

2 dessertspoons cooking oil
1 small onion, finely
    chopped
1 clove garlic, finely
    chopped
6 oz (180 g) minced beef
$\frac{1}{2}$ teaspoon Worcester
    sauce
$\frac{1}{2}$ teaspoon oregano

salt and freshly ground
    black pepper
1 small (8 oz/227 g) can of
    Italian tomatoes
4 mushrooms, sliced
2 dessertspoons tomato
    paste
2 green or red peppers,
    about 6 oz (180 g) each

Put the oil in a saucepan together with the finely
chopped onion and garlic; cook until soft and yellow but
do *not* brown. Add the minced beef, Worcester sauce,
oregano, salt and pepper. Drain the tomatoes. Put the
juice on one side. Add the tomatoes to the mixture in the
pan together with the mushrooms and tomato paste. Add
a little tomato juice if necessary to stop the mixture
sticking, but try to keep it as dry as possible. Simmer
gently for about 30 minutes, stirring frequently.

Cut the tops off the peppers and take the seeds out.
Place them in a dish where they will be kept in an upright
position. Stuff the peppers with the above mixture and
replace the tops.

Add a little water to the bottom of the dish to stop the
peppers sticking. Put in the middle of a hot oven Gas
7/425°F/220°C and cook for 25 to 35 minutes.

Kidney Mince Pie

Serves 4

4 oz (120 g) ox kidney
12 oz (360 g) raw minced
  beef
2 oz (60 g) cooking oil
2 onions, finely chopped
2 oz (60 g) plain flour
2 oz (60 g) mushrooms,
  sliced

2 medium carrots, peeled
  and grated
2 oz (60 g) frozen peas
½ pint (300 ml) stock
salt and freshly ground
  black pepper

Topping for pie
6 oz (180 g) self-raising
  flour
½ level teaspoon baking
  powder

pinch of salt
2 oz (60 g) butter
milk

Cut the kidneys into small pieces and discard all the fat and core. Mix with the mince. Put the oil in a frying pan and fry the onions until golden, *not* brown. Add the kidney and mince and continue to fry until browned, stirring all the time. Stir in the flour, then add the mushrooms, carrots, peas and stock. Season with salt and pepper. Bring to the boil and cook for a few minutes, stirring. Put the mixture into an ovenproof dish and keep warm.

For the topping: Sift together the flour and baking powder, add a pinch of salt and rub in the butter and add sufficient milk to form a soft dough. Knead lightly and roll out ½ inch thick on to a floured board. Cut into rounds with a 2-inch cutter and arrange on top of the pie in circles overlapping to cover the mince mixture. Brush with milk. Cook in the top of the oven Gas 6/400°F/200°C for approximately 30 minutes.

Lamb and Apricot Kebabs   *Serves 4*

2 tablespoons sunflower oil
1 tablespoon dry white
   wine
15½ oz (440 g) can apricot
   halves
2 oz (60 g) onion, finely
   chopped

1 clove garlic, crushed
¼ teaspoon dried thyme
bay leaves
1 lb (480 g) lean lamb
   from top of leg of lamb
salt and freshly ground
   black pepper

Make a marinade of the oil, wine, 2 tablespoons of apricot juice, onion, garlic and herbs. Cut the meat into cubes and put it in the marinade for 2 to 3 hours. Drain the apricot halves and add them to the marinade. Season with salt and freshly ground pepper. Drain meat and fruit and skewer alternately meat, fruit, bay leaf, meat, fruit, bay leaf etc. Place in grill pan and grill for about 15 minutes, turning once. Serve on a bed of boiled long grain rice.

Fillet of Lamb Dijon   *Serves 4*

4 × 4 oz (120 g) fillets of
   lamb
Dijon mustard
2 oz (60 g) butter

sunflower oil
¼ to ½ pint (150 to 300 ml)
   stock
1 bunch watercress

Trim fillets, discard all fat. Spread the mustard thickly on each side of each fillet. Melt butter in a frying pan, add a few drops of oil. Fry the fillets gently until browned on the outside and pale pink in the centre – approx. 15 to 20 minutes. Take the fillets out of the pan and place in a warm dish. Add a little stock to the juices in the pan, pour over the fillets and serve garnished with watercress.

N.B. Although a lot of mustard is used in this recipe, the finished result does not taste hot.

(Contributed by Jill F. Middleton.)

Roast Lamb with Rosemary   *Serves 4*

½ shoulder of lamb   salt and freshly ground
  (approx. 2 to   black pepper
  2½ lb/960 g to 1.2 kg)   1 clove garlic
2 tablespoons cooking oil   ½ pint (300 ml) dry white
dried rosemary   wine

Preheat oven to Gas 7/425°F/220°C. Wash and dry joint and place in a baking tin. Pour 2 tablespoons cooking oil over the joint, then sprinkle it heavily with dried rosemary, salt and black pepper. Chop the garlic very finely and add it to the wine, pour into baking tin. Roast the joint for 30 minutes in the centre of the oven at Gas 7/425°F/220°C then turn down to Gas 5/375°F/190°C and continue to cook for another 1½ hours. If it is beginning to cook too quickly, turn down to Gas 4/350°F/180°C. When ready, it should be brown with crispy fat but succulent meat.

Rosemary Lamb Casserole

Serves 6 to 8

3½ oz (105 g) butter
4 lb (1.9 kg) boned lamb
2 oz (60 g) flour
2 or 3 onions
12 oz (360 g) celery
1 lb (480 g) cooking
   apples, peeled, cored
   and sliced

1 pint (600 ml) stock
½ pint (300 ml) apple
   juice, unsweetened
salt and freshly ground
   black pepper
rosemary
1 lb (480 g) potatoes
watercress to garnish

Put 2 oz (60 g) butter with a little cooking oil in a pan and heat. Cut up the meat into small pieces, removing all fat and gristle; roll them in the flour and brown quickly in the heated fat.

Drain and put meat into a casserole dish. Slice the onions and celery finely and together with the sliced apples put them in the frying pan and fry lightly. Then put them into the casserole on top of the meat. Pour the stock and apple juice over the whole lot and season well with salt and pepper and dried rosemary.

Top with a layer of thinly sliced potatoes and dot these with butter.

Bake in a moderate oven at Gas 4/350°F/180°C for about 1½ hours. Serve garnished with watercress.

Spiced Kidneys

Serves 2

6 to 8 oz (180 to 240 g)
   lamb's kidneys
1 tablespoon flour
   seasoned with salt and
   pepper
1 tablespoon cooking oil
1 oz (30 g) butter
1 chicken stock cube

1 tablespoon white wine
   vinegar
½ teaspoon ground ginger
1 teaspoon clear honey
2 oz (60 g) sultanas
chopped fresh chives for
   garnish

Skin the kidneys and chop into pieces, discarding the cores, and toss in the seasoned flour. Heat the oil in a pan and add butter. When this begins to turn brown, quickly add the kidneys and sauté them gently for 3 minutes. Pour off half the fat and stir in the rest of the flour. Dissolve the stock cube in $\frac{1}{4}$ pint (150 ml) of hot water and add to the kidneys, stirring all the time. Add the vinegar, ginger, honey and sultanas. Bring to the boil and simmer gently for about 10 minutes.

Serve on a bed of freshly boiled long grain rice and garnish with chopped chives.

(Contributed by Jill F. Middleton.)

Savoury Liver   *Serves 2*

2 oz (60 g) butter, unsalted
1 stock cube
8 oz (240 g) sliced lamb's
    liver

chopped fresh parsley for
    garnish

Cream the butter until soft and add the crumbled stock cube. Wash and trim the liver and lay it in a grill pan without the rack. Spread half the butter mixture over the slices of liver and grill for about 10 minutes. Turn slices over after 5 minutes and spread remaining savoury butter on to the slices. Serve with the juices spooned over and garnish with chopped parsley.

(Contributed by Jill F. Middleton.)

Wiener Schnitzel

Serves 6

6 × 4 to 5 oz (120 to 150 g) slices of veal
½ wineglass of dry white wine
2 eggs
few drops water
few drops sunflower oil

3 oz (90 g) plain flour
sea salt and freshly ground black pepper
6 oz (180 g) wholewheat breadcrumbs
4 oz (120 g) butter

Trim slices and beat to flatten. Pour the white wine over the meat and leave for about an hour, turning several times. Break the eggs in a dish and mix with a few drops of oil and water. Mix the flour with the salt and pepper. Dip the marinated veal in the flour first and then into the egg mixture and finally into the breadcrumbs.

Heat the butter in the frying pan (till the flour sizzles) and fry the crumbed slices slowly until golden brown. Serve with boiled or chipped potatoes and individual side salads.

(Contributed by Jill F. Middleton.)

Baked Rabbit in Cream

Serves 4

1 rabbit
4 tablespoons French mustard
2 oz (60 g) cooking oil

6 fl.oz (180 ml) single cream
salt and freshly ground black pepper

Skin and joint rabbit. Cover the rabbit pieces thickly with the mustard. Dribble the oil over the top. Bake in a baking tin with foil over the top for 1 to 1½ hours at Gas 4/350°F/180°C.

When cooked, put the rabbit pieces on a dish and keep hot. Stir the cream into the juices over a low flame, season with salt and pepper. Cook for 2 to 3 minutes, stirring all the time. Serve the rabbit with the sauce poured over.

(Contributed by Jill F. Middleton.)

Duck with Black Cherries   *Serves 4*

4 to 5 lb (1.8 to 2.2 kg) duck, including giblets
1 small onion
2 cloves garlic
1 × 15 oz (425 g) can black cherries, stoned
4 tablespoons wholewheat breadcrumbs
3 teaspoons honey

salt and freshly ground black pepper
1 tablespoon fresh chopped sage
2 to 3 wineglasses natural apple juice
$\frac{3}{4}$ oz (20 g) cornflour
watercress, for garnish

Wash the duck and take out the giblets. Cook the giblets in a little water with salt and pepper for 10 to 15 minutes.

Meanwhile, finely chop the onion and the garlic. When the liver is cooked, take it out and mash it up with the onions and 1 clove of garlic. Take one-third of the cherries out of the can and chop them up and add to the liver mixture. Bind the stuffing together with breadcrumbs, a little of the water the giblets were cooked in, and a teaspoon of clear honey. Season with salt and freshly ground black pepper and mix in the sage.

Now stuff the duck with this mixture and put it in a roasting tin. Pour half the juice from the cherries over the duck plus a glass or two of natural apple juice and a

137

little water. Rub a spoonful of honey over the duck's skin and sprinkle liberally with salt. Prick the skin in several places with a fork. Put into a hot oven Gas 7/425°F/220°C for 30 minutes, then turn down to Gas 5/375°F/190°C and cook for another 1½ hours until the duck is brown and crispy on the outside and sweet and juicy inside, with all the fat drained off.

Meanwhile, mix the cornflour with a little of the cherry juice, then put it in a saucepan with the remainder of the cherries. Heat gently and add the remainder of the cherry juice, a teaspoon of honey and the juice from 1 crushed clove of garlic. Season with salt and black pepper. Stirring all the time, add a glass of natural apple juice. Add water if necessary to keep the sauce from getting too thick.

Serve the roast duck garnished with watercress sprigs and the sauce handed separately.

Duck with Bramble Sauce   *Serves 4*

12 oz (360 g) blackberries
2 dessert apples
2 teaspoons apple juice
2 teaspoons honey
water
4 to 5 lb (2 to 2.5 kg) duck

For the stuffing
4 oz (120 g) sage and
   onion stuffing mix
1 duck's liver
1 small onion
2 dessertspoons apple jelly
3 tablespoons bramble
   sauce
salt and pepper

Wash blackberries and put in pan. Peel and slice the apples and add to the blackberries. Add the apple juice, honey and a little water, just covering the fruit. Simmer gently. Pour off any excess juice and keep separately.

Cook until the mixture is soft and thick, with most of the juices taken up. Put on one side.

Make the stuffing mix according to the instructions on the packet. Meanwhile, cook the duck's liver in a little water. Peel and finely chop the onion and add to the stuffing mix. When the liver is cooked, chop it and add to the mixture, together with 2 dessertspoons of apple jelly and 3 tablespoons of bramble sauce. Season with salt and pepper.

Stuff the duck with the above mixture. If there is too much, put it in a dish for duck *pâté*. Sprinkle the duck with salt and pepper. Spoon 2 dessertspoons of apple jelly over it. Put in a baking pan with 3 tablespoons of apple juice. Do *not* use any fat or oil.

Put into a hot oven Gas 7/425°F/220°C for 30 minutes, then turn down to Gas 5/375°F/190°C and cook for 1½ hours until the duck is brown and crispy on the outside and sweet and succulent within. Serve with bramble sauce handed separately.

Chicken and Mushroom Pie — *Serves 4*

3 lb (1.4 kg) chicken, already cooked
1 medium onion
1 clove garlic
8 oz (240 g) mushrooms
¾ pint (450 ml) milk
chicken stock cube
4 level tablespoons plain flour
1½ oz (45 g) butter
8 oz (240 g) shortcrust pastry

Cut the chicken into chunky pieces. Finely chop the onion and garlic. Wash the mushrooms and cut them into quarters. Put the butter into a pan and gently fry the onions and mushrooms in it for 2 to 3 minutes.

Meanwhile, warm the milk in a saucepan (do not boil) and dissolve the stock cube in it.

Stir the flour into the butter which is frying the onions and mushrooms. Gradually add the milk stock, stirring all the time, until the mixture has a smooth texture.

Turn into a pie dish with a pie funnel. Allow to cool, then cover with pastry and bake in a hot oven Gas 7/425°F/220°C for 20 to 25 minutes.

Chicken Brochettes   *Serves 4*

4 × 4 oz (120 g) chicken
   breasts
2 tablespoons natural
   apple juice
1 Spanish onion
3 oz (90 g) butter
4 tablespoons chopped
   fresh parsley

salt and freshly ground
   black pepper
12 apricot halves (if dried,
   soak overnight)
black olives
1 tablespoon olive oil

Skin the chicken breasts and divide them into small mouth-sized pieces. Place on a plate and pour the natural apple juice over them. Cut the onion into chunky pieces. Beat the butter until soft and add the parsley, salt and freshly ground black pepper. Drain the apricot halves and fill the hollows with parsley butter. Drain the olives.

Thread the pieces of chicken breast, onion, stuffed apricots and olives alternately on to skewers. Brush the whole lot with a little olive oil and grill in the grill pan without a rack for about 20 minutes, turning and basting frequently. Serve with the juices spooned over.

Chicken Cassata   *Serves 4*

½ pint (300 ml) chicken
  stock
1 level tablespoon gelatine
¼ teaspoon Tabasco sauce
2 to 3 tablespoons cider
  vinegar
5 tablespoons mayonnaise
12 oz (360 g) cooked
  chicken, diced

2 teaspoons very finely
  chopped chives
2 to 3 sticks celery,
  chopped
1 small green pepper,
  diced
1 red eating apple, diced
green salad

Put the chicken stock into a saucepan, sprinkle gelatine
into it and dissolve over a low heat. Do not boil. Add the
Tabasco and cider vinegar. Leave to cool but *not* set.
Whisk the mayonnaise into the mixture gradually and
when it begins to set fold in the chicken, chives, celery,
pepper and apple. Turn into a wetted mould and leave to
set. Unmould and serve on a bed of green salad.

(Contributed by Jill F. Middleton.)

Chicken Vermouth   *Serves 4*

4 chicken breast portions
1 oz (30 g) butter
2 tablespoons sunflower oil
4 tablespoons dry
  vermouth
½ pint (300 ml) chicken
  stock
1 tablespoon fresh
  chopped tarragon

salt and freshly ground
  black pepper
8 oz (240 g) button
  mushrooms
2 level tablespoons
  cornflour
1 bunch watercress

141

Wash the joints and skin them if desired. Melt the butter in a large frying pan and add the sunflower oil. Fry the chicken portions in the mixture for about 15 minutes until they are nicely browned on both sides. Pour in the vermouth and set alight. Shake the pan gently until the flames die down. Slowly stir in the stock, tarragon and seasoning and bring to the boil. Transfer to a casserole dish with lid and cook in a medium oven Gas 4/350°F/180°C for about 40 minutes.

Wash the mushrooms and add them to the casserole, making sure they are covered by the liquid. Cook for another 10 minutes. Test the chicken to see if it is cooked. If clear liquid runs from the meat when it is spiked with a skewer, it is done. Remove the chicken pieces and put on a large serving dish. Cover with foil and keep warm. Put the juices from the casserole into a saucepan and thicken them with cornflour blended into a thin paste with a little of the juices. Boil for a few minutes, stirring continuously. Spoon over the chicken for serving and put the rest into a sauceboat. Garnish the chicken with watercress sprigs.

Chicken with Almonds   *Serves 4*

4 chicken breast portions
cooking oil
¼ pint (150 ml) chicken
   stock (can be made with
   chicken stock cube)
2 teaspoons cornflour
½ teaspoon dry mustard

3 tablespoons natural
   apple juice
½ teaspoon clear honey
2 to 3 drops Worcester
   sauce
1 oz (30 g) slivered
   almonds, toasted

Trim chicken portions and wipe clean. Arrange in a single layer in an ovenproof dish, brush with oil. Pour the chicken stock over them and bake in a medium hot oven Gas 5/375°F/190°C for about 40 minutes. Remove chicken from juice and keep warm.

Blend the cornflour and mustard with the natural apple juice, honey and Worcester sauce and stir into the bubbling juices. Keep stirring until a smooth sauce is obtained.

Place the chicken portions on a serving dish, pour the sauce over them and sprinkle the toasted almonds on top.

(Contributed by Jill F. Middleton.)

Chicken with Cashew Nuts   *Serves 4*

3½ lb (1.7 kg) whole cooked chicken
1 oz (30 g) butter
2 oz (60 g) cashews
1 medium onion, chopped
1 apple, diced
8 oz (240 g) potatoes, diced
2 teaspoons mild curry paste
½ pint (300 ml) stock made with chicken stock cube
1 to 2 oz (30 to 60 g) sultanas
salt and pepper
½ pint (300 ml) milk
2 tablespoons cream

Take the cooked meat off the chicken. Melt the butter in a pan and fry the nuts until golden brown. Add the chopped onion, diced apple and potatoes. Fry gently for about 5 minutes. Add curry paste, the meat, stock and sultanas. Cook gently for 30 minutes. Add salt and pepper to taste. Add milk slowly, stirring all the time. Add the cream just before serving.

(Contributed by Jill F. Middleton.)

Devilled Chicken   *Serves 4*

3½ lb (1.5 kg) roasting
  chicken
4 oz (120 g) plain flour
1 teaspoon barbecue spice
1 teaspoon salt
1 teaspoon paprika pepper
1 teaspoon chilli powder
1 tablespoon French
  mustard

2 tablespoons chilli sauce
2 tablespoons cider vinegar
½ teaspoon Tabasco sauce
1 egg, beaten
5 tablespoons evaporated
  milk
4 oz (120 g) butter

Joint chicken into 8 pieces. Put the flour, barbecue spice, salt, paprika pepper and chilli powder in a large bowl and mix very thoroughly.

In another bowl put the mustard, chilli sauce, cider vinegar, Tabasco, egg and evaporated milk. Mix well.

Dip each chicken portion first into the seasoned flour, then into the mustard mixture, and then again into the seasoned flour.

Melt the butter in a baking tin and arrange the chicken pieces in it, skin side down. Bake in a medium oven Gas 4/350°F/180°C for 25 minutes, then turn the pieces over, baste and bake for a further 25 minutes.

(Contributed by Jill F. Middleton.)

Grilled Chicken   *Serves 4*

4 chicken pieces
4 dessertspoons natural
  apple juice
melted butter

salt and freshly ground
  black pepper
4 tinned peaches, cut in
  halves
or 4 slices tinned pineapple

144

Sprinkle the chicken portions with the natural apple juice, then brush them with melted butter and season with salt and pepper. Preheat the grill. Place chicken portions in grill pan without the rack, ideally about 6 inches from the heat. Grill for about 10 to 12 minutes with the skin side down, then turn the pieces over skin side up and grill for a further 10 to 15 minutes. Baste with melted butter from time to time. Place 2 peach halves or one slice of pineapple on each chicken portion for the last 5 minutes' grilling, and spoon a little of the fruit syrup over each. Serve with green salad and jacket potatoes.

(Contributed by Jill F. Middleton.)

Italian Chicken Breasts
Serves 4

1 tablespoon cooking oil
4 chicken breasts
1 lb (480 g) potatoes, peeled
6 oz (180 g) button mushrooms
6 oz (180 g) onion, chopped
16 stuffed olives
3 tablespoons dry white vermouth
2 tablespoons tomato paste
2 level tablespoons cornflour
1 level teaspoon dried oregano
$\frac{3}{4}$ pint (450 ml) chicken stock (can be made with chicken stock cube)

Heat the cooking oil in a large pan and lightly fry the chicken breasts until brown on both sides. Drain and place them in an ovenproof casserole dish. Cut the potatoes into small fingers. Wash but do not peel the mushrooms. Put the potatoes, mushrooms and chopped onion in the pan and fry until golden brown. Then add these to the chicken in the casserole. Sprinkle the stuffed olives over the top.

Add the white vermouth, tomato paste, cornflour and oregano to the stock and mix well. Pour over the chicken. Put a lid on the casserole and cook in a moderate oven, Gas 4/350°F/180°C, until tender, which will be in 45 minutes to 1 hour.

Mexican Chicken in the Brick   *Serves 4*

1 × 3½ lb (1.7 kg) chicken
1 packet American savoury
   rice
1 clove garlic
1 small apple
1 small onion
clear honey
1 teaspoon ground ginger

2 dessertspoons curry
   powder
1 tablespoon peanuts or
   cashew nuts
2 tablespoons sultanas
1 knob butter
salt and pepper
cooking oil

Wash the chicken, take out the giblets and use for stock. Cook the savoury rice according to the instructions on the packet. Meanwhile, finely chop the onion, garlic and apple. Add these to the cooked rice, plus a dessertspoon of honey, the ground ginger and curry powder. For those who like hot curries, add extra curry powder. Mix in the nuts and sultanas. Add a knob of butter. Now stuff this mixture into the chicken until it is quite full. Place the chicken in a chicken brick. Dribble a little cooking oil over it, plus a teaspoon of clear honey. Sprinkle liberally with curry powder and a little salt and pepper. If you have any of the stuffing mixture left over, put it round the chicken at the bottom of the brick and sprinkle with curry powder and a few drops of oil and honey.

Put into a cold oven set at Gas 9/470°F/240°C, and cook for 1½ to 2 hours. Serve with a tossed green salad.

Roast Chicken with Peaches   *Serves 4*

1 × 3½ lb (1.7 kg) chicken,   salt and freshly ground
   including giblets   black pepper
6 oz (180 g) wholewheat   1 × 15 oz (425 g) tin
   breadcrumbs   peaches in syrup, sliced
1 small onion, finely   2 teaspoons honey
   chopped   2 tablespoons cooking oil
1 rasher gammon bacon
   (optional)

Wash the chicken and remove the giblets. Put the giblets in a pan with salt and pepper and boil gently for 20 minutes.

Put the breadcrumbs in a bowl and mix in the finely chopped onion. If you use bacon, add it finely chopped. Remove the chicken liver from the pan and mash it up and add it to the mixture in the bowl. Season with salt and freshly ground black pepper.

Drain the peaches, add them to the mixture together with a tablespoon of the syrup from the tin and a teaspoon of honey. Make the mixture damp enough for it to stick together, adding more peach syrup if necessary. Stuff the chicken with this mixture and put it in a roasting tin. Rub a teaspoon of honey over the skin, sprinkling liberally with salt and pepper. Pour the remainder of the peach syrup over, then add the cooking oil. Roast the chicken in a hot oven, Gas 7/425°F/220°C, for 30 minutes. Turn down to Gas 5/375°F/190°C and continue to cook for another hour. Baste frequently.

For a change, add a piece of stem ginger, finely chopped, from a jar of stem ginger in syrup. Pour a little of the ginger syrup over the peaches.

Polynesian Chicken

4 chicken portions
2 tablespoons cooking oil
15 oz (425 g) can
   pineapple chunks
1 tablespoon soy sauce
2 or 3 sticks celery,
   chopped

1 level tablespoon
   cornflour
3 tablespoons water
2 tomatoes or 1 red pepper
1 green pepper

Trim and dry chicken portions. Put the oil in a pan and brown the chicken pieces on both sides. Drain chicken and keep warm. Drain pineapple and make juice up to $\frac{1}{4}$ pint (150 ml) with water, if necessary. Add pineapple juice and soy sauce to the pan. Stir in chopped celery and simmer for 20 minutes. Blend cornflour with the 3 tablespoons water and stir into the mixture in the pan. Bring to the boil. Add pineapple chunks. Cut tomatoes into 8 wedges or, if using red pepper, cut into rings and add to the mixture. Cut green pepper into rings, discard seeds and add to pan. Place chicken portions on top and simmer for a further 10 to 15 minutes until the chicken is tender. Serve with rice.

(Contributed by Jill F. Middleton.)

Spiced Chicken Drumsticks

2 to 3 chicken legs per
   person
2 dessertspoons curry
   powder

cooking oil
clear honey
salt

Wash the chicken legs and dry them. Mix the curry powder with a little cooking oil, then roll each leg in the mixture until it is completely covered. Arrange the chicken legs in a grill pan without the grid and dribble clear honey over them. Sprinkle with salt. Grill for 10 to 15 minutes until they are crisp on the outside. They will go a very dark brown and the honey makes them burn easily. Serve with rice or bread and a mixed salad.

Sweet and Sour Chicken *Serves 4*

2 tablespoons sunflower oil
4 chicken breasts
½ pint (300 ml) chicken
  stock
8 oz (227 g) can of
  pineapple pieces
2 oz (60 g) green pepper,
  sliced
2 oz (60 g) red pepper,
  sliced

¼ teaspoon chilli powder
2 tablespoons cornflour
1 tablespoon soy sauce
8 tablespoons white wine
  vinegar
1 level tablespoon
  molasses or black
  treacle

Put the oil in a pan and fry the chicken in it until brown. Drain the chicken and put in a casserole dish. Pour the chicken stock over (this can be made with a stock cube). Put a lid on the casserole and cook in a moderate oven, Gas 4/350°F/180°C, for about 45 minutes.

Pour the juices off into a saucepan. Keep the chicken pieces hot. Add the pineapple and green and red peppers to the stock in the saucepan and simmer for 5 minutes. Add the chilli powder to the cornflour and blend with the soy sauce, vinegar and treacle. Add to the stock, stirring all the time until the sauce thickens and becomes transparent. Add salt and pepper to taste.

Pour the sauce over the chicken pieces and serve on a bed of freshly-boiled Patna rice.

(Contributed by Jill F. Middleton.)

149

Partridge with Grapes

Serves 2

2 young partridges
2 tablespoons sunflower oil
6 fl. oz (180 ml) stock (can
   be made with a chicken
   stock cube)
6 tablespoons dry white
   wine
salt and freshly ground
   black pepper

4 oz (120 g) white grapes
1 level tablespoon
   cornflour
1 egg yolk
2 tablespoons double
   cream
chopped parsley, for
   garnish

Cut the partridges in half and remove the backbones and the outside skin. Put the oil in a pan and lightly fry the partridge halves in it until they are golden brown on both sides. Now pour the stock and wine over the birds and season with the salt and freshly ground black pepper. Bring the mixture to the boil and simmer gently for about 25 minutes until the meat is tender.

Meanwhile, wash the grapes, cut them in halves and remove the pips. Blend together the cornflour, egg yolk and cream. When the partridges are cooked, take them out of the pan, drain them and keep them warm on a serving dish.

Add the cornflour mixture and the grapes to the juices in the pan. Cook gently without boiling until the sauce thickens. Stir frequently. Add seasoning if necessary. Pour the sauce over the partridge halves, garnish with the parsley and serve immediately.

N.B. The same recipe can be used for pigeons.

Turkey Breasts in Sour Cream   *Serves 4*

1 lb (480 g) turkey breasts
2 tablespoons sunflower oil
3 oz (90 g) onions finely
  chopped
2 level teaspoons ground
  paprika
¾ pint (450 ml) stock (can
  be made with a chicken
  stock cube)
1 green pepper, seeded
  and sliced in strips

4 oz (120 g) small pasta
  shapes
salt and freshly ground
  black pepper
¼ pint (150 ml) carton
  soured cream
1 level teaspoon cornflour
fresh parsley, chopped, for
  garnish

Skin the turkey breasts if necessary and cut them into
small strips. Heat the oil in a pan and gently fry the
chopped onion until golden brown. Add the turkey and
paprika to the pan. Stir and fry quickly to seal the turkey
pieces. Stir in the stock and bring to the boil. Add the
pieces of green pepper and pasta and season with salt
and pepper.

Put a lid on the pan and simmer gently for 15 to 20
minutes until the turkey and pasta are tender. Stir in the
soured cream and thicken with the blended cornflour.
Serve garnished with chopped parsley.

Spiced Turkey *Serves 4*

4 turkey wings
3 oz (90 g) stem ginger
1 × 15 oz (425 g) can of
   pineapple pieces
8 tablespoons soy sauce
3 tablespoons dry white
   wine vinegar
8 tablespoons dry white
   wine

Angostura bitters
2 tablespoons ginger syrup
   from jar
salt and freshly ground
   black pepper
spring onions and chives,
   chopped, to garnish

Joint the turkey wings, discard the pinions and take off the skin. Make cuts in the flesh so that the meat absorbs the marinade.

Place the turkey wings in a shallow ovenproof dish in one layer. Slice the ginger into small strips and mix with the drained pineapple pieces. Add the soy sauce, wine vinegar, white wine, a few drops of Angostura bitters and ginger syrup, and mix well. Season with salt and pepper and spoon the whole mixture over the turkey. Cover and marinate overnight.

Next day, cook in a covered dish in a hot oven, Gas 7/425°F/220°C, for about 1 hour until the flesh is tender. Baste as necessary. Serve garnished with finely chopped onions and chives.

Chicken can be cooked the same way, but you will need to allow more chicken per person than turkey.

15

Desserts

Almond and Apricot Lattice   *Serves 4*

3½ oz (105 g) butter
7 oz (210 g) plain flour
2 oz (60 g) castor sugar
2 oz (60 g) ground
  almonds
3 egg yolks

1 lb (480 g) apricots
  (dried apricots may be
  used but be sure to soak
  them overnight)
2 tablespoons icing sugar

Rub the butter into the sifted flour and add castor sugar and ground almonds. Bind together with the beaten egg yolks and a little cold water. Roll this out and line an 8-in (200-mm) flan tin with it.

Halve and stone the apricots (if using fresh) and arrange them in the flan case. Sprinkle with the sifted icing sugar.

Use remaining pastry mixture to make a lattice over the apricots.

Bake in a moderate oven at Gas 5/375° F/190° C for about 30 minutes. Sprinkle with icing sugar before serving.

Almond Fingers *Serves 4*

8 oz (240 g) shortcrust
  pastry
apricot jam
1 egg white
3 oz (90 g) ground
  almonds
3 oz (90 g) castor sugar

2 teaspoons ground rice
1 oz (30 g) almonds,
  chopped and skinned
few drops almond essence
6 to 7 in (152 to 178 mm)
  square tin

Grease the tin and line it with pastry. Spread the jam (which should be fairly runny) over the pastry, not too thickly. Whisk the egg white well and fold in the rest of the ingredients. Spread this mixture over the jam. Bake in a moderate oven, Gas 4 to 5/350° to 375° F/180° to 190° C, for about 25 minutes. When nearly cool, cut into fingers and finish cooling on a wire tray.

(Contributed by Mrs J. R. Wentworth.)

Apple Cheesecake *Serves 6*

2 oz (60 g) digestive
  biscuits, finely crushed
2 oz (60 g) muesli, dry
2 oz (60 g) butter
1 oz (30 g) soft brown
  muscovado sugar
8 oz (240 g) cream cheese
5 fl. oz (150 ml) sour
  cream
2 egg yolks

2 teaspoons clear honey
$\frac{1}{2}$ oz (15 g) gelatine
4 tablespoons water
2 egg whites
$1\frac{1}{2}$ oz (45 g) clear honey
1 red apple
2 oz (60 g) seedless grapes
walnut halves
2 tablespoons clear honey

Grease an 8-in (200-mm) flan tin. Mix the crushed biscuits and dry muesli together. Melt the butter in a pan and add the biscuit mixture and the brown sugar. Stir well. Press this firmly over the bottom of the tin and place in the refrigerator for 10 to 15 minutes.

Meanwhile, beat the cream cheese and sour cream together, gradually adding the egg yolks and 2 teaspoons of honey. Beat until a smooth texture is obtained.

Dissolve the gelatine in 2 tablespoons water. When it is cool but not set, stir it into the cheese mixture. Whisk the egg whites, gradually adding the 1½ oz (45 g) honey. Beat until it makes peaks, then gently fold into the cheese mixture. Pour into the prepared tin and chill until set.

Decorate the top of the cake with unpeeled sliced apples, seedless grapes and walnut halves. Make a glaze with the remaining honey dissolved in a little water and brush over the apples and grapes.

Cinnamon Apple Jelly *Serves 6*

2 lb (960 g) apples
½ pint (300 ml) water
½ pint (300 ml) natural
  apple juice
4 oz (120 g) clear honey
2 cloves

1½ oz (45 g) gelatine
4 tablespoons cold water
1 egg
2 teaspoons ground
  cinnamon

Peel and core apples, and cook with the water, apple juice, honey and cloves until soft.

Soak gelatine in the 4 tablespoons cold water for a few minutes, then heat until dissolved. Beat the egg and keep on one side.

Sieve the apples. Strain gelatine and stir into apple purée. Add 1 teaspoon of the cinnamon and fold in the beaten egg.

Pour into serving dish and leave to set. Before serving, sprinkle top with the rest of the cinnamon.

Apricot Cheesecake *Serves 6*

1 lb (450 g) dried apricots
3½ oz (105 g) clear honey
4 oz (120 g) digestive
  biscuits
6 oz (180 g) butter
1 level teaspoon ground
  mixed spice
4 level teaspoons
  powdered gelatine

½ wineglass dry white
  wine
8 oz (240 g) carton
  cottage cheese
8 oz (240 g) carton cream
  cheese
1 × 14 oz (397 g) tin
  evaporated milk

Soak the apricots overnight in cold water. Simmer them in 7 fl. oz (210 ml) water plus 2 oz (60 g) honey for about 20 minutes until cooked. Crumble biscuits half at a time, in grinder or by hand. Put into a bowl and mix with the butter which you have previously melted, mixed spice and 1½ oz (45 g) honey.

Use three-quarters of the crumbs to line the base of an 8½-in (210-mm) spring release mould. Refrigerate to set.

Dissolve the gelatine in the wine and put it in the blender together with the cheese and evaporated milk. Blend until smooth. Put into separate bowl and fold in the roughly chopped apricots. Pour mixture into crumb case, scatter the rest of the biscuit crumbs on top and refrigerate to set. Turn out upside down and serve. It can be dredged with icing sugar, if desired, or decorated with apricots saved from the chopped ones.

Apricot Kuchen *Serves 4 to 6*

8 oz (240 g) rich
  shortcrust pastry
3 egg whites
4 oz (120 g) ground
  almonds

1 lb (480 g) fresh apricots
4 fl. oz (120 ml) double
  cream
4 fl. oz (120 ml) clear
  honey syrup

Grease a 10-in (255-mm) flan tin, and line the tin with the pastry. Whisk egg whites till firm and fold in the ground almonds. Spread this mixture on to the pastry.

Cut apricots in half and remove stones. Arrange apricots, cut side up, on top of almond mixture. Bake in a hot oven Gas 6 or 7/400 to 425° F/200 to 220° C for 10 minutes, then reduce heat to Gas 4/350° F/180° C and cook for a further 45 minutes until the pastry is cooked.

Serve warm. Whip the cream and hand separately with clear honey syrup (melted honey).

(Contributed by Jill F. Middleton.)

Apricot Sorbet *Serves 6*

6 oz (180 g) dried apricots
3 oz (90 g) soft brown
  muscovado sugar

3 tablespoons natural
  apple juice
1 egg white

Place the apricots in water to soak overnight, then poach them in the liquid in which they have soaked for about 45 minutes, using a covered pan.

Strain off the liquid and make up to $\frac{1}{2}$ pint (300 ml) with water, return to the pan and add the brown sugar. Bring to the boil and keep boiling for 2 to 3 minutes. Allow to cool, then blend the apricots with a little of the syrup and the natural apple juice. This is best done in a blender. Stir the rest of the liquid into the purée and freeze the mixture until it is a mushy consistency.

Put the mushy mixture into a cold bowl and beat well until it is of a smooth texture. Fold in the stiffly-whisked egg white and return to the freezer. Freeze until firm. Transfer to the refrigerator for about an hour before serving.

Apricot Whip   *Serves 4*

$\frac{1}{4}$ pint (150 ml) apricot
  purée (preferably made
  from fresh apricots)
1$\frac{1}{2}$ oz (45 g) clear honey
2 egg whites

5 fl. oz (150 ml) carton
  whipping cream
$\frac{1}{4}$ pint (150 ml) water
1 dessertspoon vodka
1 teaspoon almond
  essence

Put the apricot purée in a pan and heat. Add the honey and stir until dissolved, keeping the purée simmering all the time.

Beat the egg whites until stiff. Pour the purée over the egg whites and beat the two together for a couple of minutes until it is quite thick. Leave to cool.

Whip the cream until it peaks and fold it into the mixture when it is cold. Stir in the vodka, almond essence and water. Pour into serving dishes and chill.

Aromatic Fruit Salad

Serves 4

½ teaspoon clear honey
pinch allspice
1 tablespoon water
24 to 30 grapes
1 medium eating apple
8 dried apricots

1 oz (30 g) preserved
  dates
4 peaches
1 wineglass apple juice,
  unsweetened
flaked almonds, to
  decorate

Simmer honey and allspice in the water. Cool. Halve grapes and remove pips. Core and chop apple, including skin. Chop dried apricots and dates. Slice peaches. Put all the fruit, allspice, honey mixture and apple juice in a bowl and leave to soak so that the apricots soften. More apple juice can be added if needed. Sprinkle with flaked almonds before serving.

Blackberry and Pear Tarts

Serves 6

8 oz (240 g) plain flour
2 tcaspoons clear honey
3 oz (90 g) butter
1 egg
few drops vanilla essence
¼ pint (150 ml) water
3 oz (90 g) clear honey

2 pears, approx. 8 oz
  (240 g) or 1 × 15 oz
  (425 g) can of pears
8 oz (240 g) blackberries
3 oz (90 g) cream cheese
3 oz (90 g) soft brown
  muscovado sugar
1 tablespoon milk
2 teaspoons arrowroot

Sift the flour into a bowl and add 2 teaspoons clear honey and the butter. Mix together and then add the lightly-beaten egg and vanilla essence. Knead well until

159

it becomes a dough then put in a cool place for 30 minutes.

Take 6 individual flan tins and grease them. Roll the pastry out to about a quarter of an inch (6 mm) and cut out rounds to fit each flan tin and make a pastry case. Line each case with metal foil. Bake the cases blind at Gas 6/400° F/200° C for 8 to 10 minutes. Remove foil and allow to cool.

Meanwhile put the water and 3 oz (90 g) honey into a saucepan, and heat until it becomes syrup. Peel and core the pears and gently poach them in the syrup for about 30 minutes or until they are tender. Remove from the heat and add the blackberries. Cover the pan and allow to cool.

Put the cream cheese, brown sugar and milk into a bowl and beat until they form a soft creamy consistency. Cover the base of each tartlet with the cream cheese mixture and top this with the drained fruit.

Blend the arrowroot with the fruit juice in a small pan, until smooth. Bring to the boil, gently stirring all the time. Take off the heat when the sauce has thickened and cleared. When cool, use it to glaze the fruit in the tartlets.

Bramble Fool (Blackberry)   *Serves 4 to 6*

2 dessert apples
1 lb (480 g) blackberries
1 tablespoon water
3 oz (90 g) honey

2 tablespoons custard
  powder
$\frac{1}{2}$ pint (300 ml) milk
$\frac{1}{4}$ pint (150 ml) whipping
  cream

Peel and core the apples and chop into small pieces. Wash the blackberries. Put the apples and blackberries

160

in a saucepan with the water and pour the honey over it. Put a lid on the pan and simmer until the fruit is soft. Allow to cool. Blend the mixture into a purée in a blender or mash it through a sieve.

Put the custard powder into a saucepan with 2 tablespoons of the milk. Mix well and then add the remainder of the milk. Bring the mixture to the boil, stirring all the time. Remove from the stove and stir in the bramble purée, pour into a serving dish. Now whip the cream until stiff and lightly marble it into the fool.

Serve with crisp digestive biscuits.

Blackcurrant Ice Cream   *Serves 4*

1 × 6 fl. oz (170 ml) can
   evaporated milk
⅓ bottle (11.5 fl. oz/326
   ml) blackcurrant juice

Whip evaporated milk and mix in the blackcurrant juice. Put into dish and cover with foil.

Freeze for 2 hours in ice compartment of refrigerator or deep freeze. Stir the mixture thoroughly every 30 minutes.

(Contributed by Jill F. Middleton.)

Blackcurrant Lattice   *Serves 4 to 6*

6 oz (180 g) shortcrust pastry	1 level dessertspoon ground cinnamon
8 oz (240 g) blackcurrants	brown muscovado sugar
¼ pint (150 ml) water	1 egg white

Line a pie plate with about two-thirds of the pastry. Roll out the remainder of the pastry and cut in strips for the lattice.

Put the blackcurrants into a saucepan with the water and cinnamon. Simmer gently until tender. Add the brown sugar to taste. Cook a little longer until slightly reduced. Allow to cool, then pour into the pie dish.

Cover with the strips forming a lattice. Brush with egg white and sprinkle brown sugar over the top. Bake in a medium oven, Gas 6/400° F/200° C, until pastry is browned, about 25 to 30 minutes. Serve with custard or single cream.

(Contributed by Jill F. Middleton.)

Cherry Almond Tarts   *Serves 2*

4 oz (120 g) plain flour   1 oz (30 g) clear honey
2 oz (60 g) ground   ¼ pint (150 ml) water
  almonds   2 teaspoons cornflour
1 oz (30 g) castor sugar   2 tablespoons Kirsch
3 oz (90 g) butter   1 oz (30 g) almonds,
8 oz (240 g) red cherries   chopped

Make an almond pastry with the plain flour, ground almonds, castor sugar and butter.

Use two-thirds of the pastry to line 2 × 4-in (102-mm) flan tins. Make thin strips out of the remaining pastry and keep on one side.

Stone the cherries and cook with the honey and water until tender. Drain well and keep the juices on one side.

Blend the cornflour with the Kirsch and stir into the fruit juice. Bring the mixture to the boil, stirring all the time. Add the cherries and chopped almonds. Allow to

162

cool, then spoon into the pastry cases. Use the pastry strips to make a lattice covering over each tart. Bake in a moderate oven, Gas 6/400° F/200° C, for 20 to 25 minutes.

Leave to cool before removing from tins.

Cherry Ginger Jelly   *Serves 6*

1 × 5 oz (142 g) packet red jelly
2 or 3 peaches

¼ pint (150 ml) boiling water
1 lb (480 g) black cherries

½ to ¾ pint (300 to 450 ml) ginger ale
¼ pint (150 ml) whipping cream

2 teaspoons preserved stem ginger, chopped

Dissolve the jelly in the ¼ pint (150 ml) boiling water. Make up to 1 pint with ginger ale.

Skin peaches, remove stones and slice finely. Wash and stone cherries. When the jelly has set to the consistency of unbeaten egg white, fold in the sliced peaches and cherries. Pour into a wetted 2-pint (1-l) ring mould and allow to set.

Meanwhile whisk the cream until stiff and fold in the chopped ginger. When the jelly is set, turn out on to a serving dish and fill the centre with the whipped cream mixture.

(Contributed by Jill F. Middleton.)

Cherry Tart

Serves 4 to 6

6 oz (180 g) shortcrust
  pastry
1½ oz (45 g) clear honey
2 level tablespoons plain
  flour

¼ level teaspoon cinnamon
1 × 15 oz (425 g) can
  black cherries
1 oz (30 g) butter

Roll out two-thirds of the pastry and line a 7-in (178-mm) pie plate. Put the honey, flour, cinnamon and ¼ pint (150 ml) of the cherry juice from the tin into a saucepan and cook gently until the mixture thickens and boils.

Meanwhile drain the cherries. Pour the mixture from the pan over the cherries and allow to cool a little before piling it into the pastry case. Dot with butter. Roll out the rest of the pastry and use to cover the pie. Seal the edges and make 2 or 3 slits through the pastry. Bake until browned in a hot oven, Gas 7/425° F/220° C, for 35 to 45 minutes.

(Contributed by Jill F. Middleton.)

Compote of Gooseberries

Serves 4

1 lb (480 g) gooseberries
2 oz (60 g) clear honey
½ pint (300 ml) water

1 tablespoon apricot jam
2 tablespoons Kirsch

Top and tail the gooseberries. Blanch for 2 minutes in boiling water. Strain and put on one side. Boil the honey in ½ pint (300 ml) water for 10 minutes, then add the jam, Kirsch and strained gooseberries. Simmer gently until the fruit is soft. Strain the gooseberries and put them into a serving dish. Continue to simmer the remaining juice until it becomes a syrup, then pour it over the fruit. Chill thoroughly. Serve with sponge fingers handed separately.

(Contributed by Jill F. Middleton.)

Gooseberry Cream   *Serves 4 to 6*

1½ lb (720 g) gooseberries
¼ pint (150 ml) water
honey
2 oz (60 g) unsalted butter

3 eggs, beaten
1 to 2 dessertspoons
orange flower water
(optional)

Top and tail the gooseberries and put them in a saucepan with the water. Cook slowly, until soft, then put them through a sieve, or purée them in a blender. Approximately 1 pint (600 ml) of purée is needed. Sweeten with honey and reheat.

Add the butter and beaten eggs, stirring continuously over a low heat, until the mixture is a thick creamy consistency. Do *not* let it boil or the eggs will curdle. Flavour with the orange flower water, or alternatively put a head of elderflowers tied in muslin into the mixture after adding the eggs and butter and remove it when the flavour is right. It should add just a very delicate flavour. Leave to cool.

Serve in sundae glasses.

165

Gooseberry Fool *Serves 4*

1 lb (480 g) gooseberries
6 level tablespoons thick
  honey
2 level tablespoons
  powdered gelatine

4 fl. oz (120 ml) whipping
  cream
1 oz (30 g) walnuts,
  chopped

Wash the gooseberries and top and tail them. Put them in a saucepan with ¼ pint (150 ml) of water and the honey and cook until soft. While they are cooking, soak the gelatine in 2 tablespoons of water in a small jug.

Blend the fruit and juice together with the soaked gelatine (this is best done in a blender). Sieve to remove the seeds and leave to cool.

Whip the cream and fold it into the cooled purée. Turn into 4 glass dishes and refrigerate to set. When set, sprinkle the chopped walnuts on top.

Gooseberry Tart *Serves 4 to 6*

8 oz (240 g) shortcrust
  pastry
1½ lb (720 g) gooseberries,
  topped and tailed

½ pint (300 ml) single
  cream
1½ oz (45 g) clear honey
2 egg yolks

Line a large flan tin or small tart tins with the pastry. Arrange the gooseberries close together in a single layer on top of the pastry. Mix the cream, honey and egg yolks together and pour over the gooseberries.

Bake in a moderate oven, Gas 6/400° F/200° C, for 30 minutes for one large tart, or 15 minutes if using small tart tins. Serve warm or cold.

Wiltshire Gooseberry Pudding   *Serves 4 to 6*

4 oz (120 g) plain flour   soft brown muscovado
2 eggs   sugar
½ pint (300 ml) milk   butter
1 lb (480 g) gooseberries

Make a batter mix with the plain flour, 2 eggs and a scant ½ pint (300 ml) milk. Leave it to stand for 30 minutes.

Top and tail the gooseberries and three-quarters fill a 2-pint (1-l) basin. Pour the batter over the fruit, cover the basin with a cloth and steam the pudding for about an hour, or until done.

Serve with a dish of fresh butter and a dish of brown sugar to help yourself. Mix with the pudding on your plate.

(Contributed by Jill F. Middleton.)

Fresh Peach Ice Cream   *Serves 6*

12 oz (360 g) fresh   ¼ pint (150 ml) carton
   skinned peaches   whipping cream
1 × 14 oz (397 g) can   1 fresh peach
   condensed milk   flaked almonds
3 tablespoons natural
   apple juice

Slice the peaches, discarding the stones, and put them into the blender with the condensed milk, natural apple juice and cream. Blend until the mixture is quite smooth and very creamy. Pour into ice trays or a shallow polythene container and freeze until firm.

Take out of freezer and put in refrigerator for 30 minutes before serving. Decorate with slices of fresh peach and flaked almonds, and serve.

Chestnut Pears
Serves 4 to 6

1 × 1 lb 13 oz (822 g) can pear halves
1 tube sweetened chestnut purée

4 fl. oz (120 ml) whipped cream
2 oz (60 g) mixed nuts, chopped

Drain the pears and arrange the halves on a serving dish. Fill the centres with the chestnut purée. Top with whipped cream and sprinkle the chopped nuts over the top.

Pineapple Custards
Serves 4

2 × 15 oz (425 g) cans pineapple pieces
1 oz (30 g) trifle sponge cake, broken in pieces
1 whole egg
1 egg yolk

5 fl. oz (150 ml) carton whipping cream
5 tablespoons milk
2 tablespoons soft brown muscovado sugar

Crush the pineapple pieces and put a little in each of 4 small soufflé dishes. Then divide the sponge amongst the four. Beat the whole egg and add the extra yolk. Add the cream and milk, beat until smooth.

Pour the mixture into the dishes. Put the dishes in a baking tin half filled with water. Bake in a warm oven, Gas 3/325° F/170° C, for 30 to 35 minutes until set. Chill well and serve sprinkled with the brown sugar.

168

Pineapple Delight
Serves 4

6 to 8 macaroon biscuits
1 × 15 oz (425 g) can
  pineapple pieces
$\frac{1}{4}$ pint (150 ml) evaporated
  milk

$\frac{1}{2}$ pint (300 ml) cold thick
  custard
ratafia biscuits

Crush the macaroons and put in a bowl. Crush the pineapple pieces and drain them. Cover the macaroons with a layer of the crushed pineapple. Whip the evaporated milk and add it to the cold custard, whip again thoroughly, then fold in the rest of the crushed pineapple.

Pile this mixture on to the macaroons and serve decorated with ratafia biscuits.

Pineapple Upside-Down Pudding
Serves 4

2 tablespoons clear honey
12 slices pineapple
4 oz (120 g) cake crumbs
2 oz (60 g) ground
  almonds

4 tablespoons milk
2 oz (60 g) Barbados sugar
2 eggs
2 oz (60 g) butter

Line a 7-in (178-mm) square tin with greased grease-proof paper. Put the honey on the bottom and arrange pineapple slices on top of this, putting a couple of slices on one side to chop up.

Put the cake crumbs and ground almonds in a bowl, pour on the milk and the chopped pineapple. Separate the eggs. Cream the butter and sugar and beat in the egg yolks, then add the almond mixture. Beat the egg whites until stiff, then fold them into the mixture.

Bake for 30 to 40 minutes in a moderately hot oven, Gas 4 to 5/350° to 375° F/180° to 190° C. Turn out and serve.

Prune Mousse *Serves 4*

8 oz (240 g) dried prunes
3 tablespoons natural
  apple juice
2 level teaspoons
  powdered gelatine

2 level teaspoons clear
  honey
$\frac{1}{4}$ pint (150 ml) whipping
  cream
1 egg white
flaked almonds, to decorate

Soak the prunes in cold water overnight. Put prunes in a saucepan, cover them with the liquid they have been soaking in and simmer with the lid on until tender, approx. 20 minutes.

Soak gelatine in a small basin with 3 tablespoons natural apple juice. Drain the prunes, saving $\frac{1}{4}$ pint (150 ml) of the liquid. Stone them and put them in the blender with the $\frac{1}{4}$ pint (150 ml) juice, gelatine mixture and honey and blend until smooth.

In separate bowls, whip the cream and egg white until stiff. Fold the cream into the blended mixture, then fold in the beaten egg white. Refrigerate to set and decorate with flaked almonds.

Strawberry Foam

Serves 4

8 oz (240 g) fresh
  strawberries
1 tablespoon clear honey
¼ pint (150 ml) water

1 packet strawberry
  flavoured jelly
1 × 14.5 oz (410 g) can
  evaporated milk

Wash and hull the strawberries. Cut up half of them and cook them with the honey in ¼ pint (150 ml) of water until soft. Dissolve the jelly in the hot mixture, then blend to a purée. Pour into a bowl and leave to cool until partially set.

Whisk the evaporated milk until thick and creamy, then gradually whisk into the partially-set jelly. Whisk whole mixture well, and pour into serving dish or dishes and leave to set.

When completely set, decorate with the remainder of the fresh strawberries.

Strawberry Ice Pudding

Serves 6

½ pint (300 ml) custard
1 oz (30 g) clear honey
1 pint (600 ml) crushed
  strawberries
½ pint (300 ml) whipping
  cream
cochineal (optional)

For decoration
whipped cream
pineapple chunks
tinned or glacé cherries

Add the custard and honey to the crushed strawberries. Whip the cream and fold it into the strawberry mixture. If required, add a little cochineal to enhance the colour.

Put into container and freeze quickly, stirring from time to time. When set but not completely hard, press into a 2-pint (1-1) *bombe* mould. Put a layer of greaseproof paper under the lid. Seal the join with lard. Refreeze.

To serve, ease out on to a chilled serving dish and decorate with whipped cream, pineapple chunks and cherries.

Strawberry Shortcakes   *Serves 6*

8 oz (240 g) plain flour
2 teaspoons baking
  powder
2 oz (60 g) butter
1 oz (30 g) soft brown
  muscovado sugar

1 egg
12 oz (360 g) strawberries
castor sugar
¼ pint (150 ml) whipping
  cream

Sieve flour and baking powder into a bowl. Rub in the butter and add the soft brown sugar. Mix in the egg and a little milk if necessary until a stiff dough is obtained. Roll out to an inch (25 mm) thick. Cut into rounds 3 in (76 mm) diameter, and place on a greased baking sheet. Bake in a hot oven, Gas 7/425° F/220° C, for 7 to 10 minutes until well risen and browned.

Meanwhile, mash the strawberries and sweeten to taste with a little castor sugar. In a separate bowl, beat the cream until thick and stiff.

When the shortcakes are cooked, split in half while still hot and sandwich them together with crushed strawberries. Place more strawberries plus the whipped cream on top.

(Contributed by Jill F. Middleton.)

'Chocolate' Fudge

Serves 6

2 oz (60 g) butter
2 tablespoons carob
  powder
1 lb (480 g) raw sugar or
  soft brown muscovado
  sugar

$\frac{1}{4}$ pint (150 ml) milk
$\frac{1}{2}$ teaspoon vanilla essence

Put the butter in a saucepan and when it has melted add the carob powder. Stir well and add the sugar and the milk. Heat gently until the sugar is dissolved, stirring all the time. Bring the mixture to the boil and let it continue to boil until the mixture forms a soft ball when a drop is placed in a bowl of cold water (237° F/115° C).

Remove from heat and add the vanilla essence. Let the mixture cool slightly then beat it until it is thick. Pour it into a prepared greased tin and leave to set. When cold, cut into squares.

'Chocolate' Pudding

Serves 6

1$\frac{1}{2}$ oz (45 g) carob powder
4 fl. oz (120 ml) boiling
  water
3 dessertspoons cornflour
4 oz (120 g) dried milk
  powder

pinch salt
1 tablespoon clear honey
1 pint (600 ml) cold water
3 egg yolks
1 teaspoon vanilla essence

Put the carob powder in a small bowl, and stir in the 4 fl. oz (120 ml) of boiling water, keeping the mixture smooth. Leave to stand on one side.

Mix the cornflour and dried milk powder together,

173

add a pinch of salt and a tablespoon of honey. Gradually add the cold water and whisk well so that all the ingredients are blended.

Put the mixture in a double boiler over hot water and heat until the pudding thickens, stirring continuously. Cook for another 10 to 15 minutes.

Beat the egg yolks and then blend them into the pudding mixture. Cook for a few more minutes.

Remove double boiler from the heat and add the vanilla essence. Pour the mixture into a serving dish and allow to cool. Chill in a refrigerator and serve with whipped cream.

Ice Cream with Hot 'Chocolate' Sauce   *Serves 4*

1 family block vanilla
  ice cream
2 to 4 oz (60 to 120 g)
  chopped nuts or flaked
  almonds

For the sauce
1 oz (30 g) butter
1 heaped tablespoon carob
  powder
$\frac{1}{4}$ oz (7 g) cornflour
$\frac{1}{2}$ pint (300 ml) water
1 teaspoon Tia Maria
  (optional)
a few drops vanilla essence

Melt the butter in a saucepan and stir in the carob powder. Blend the cornflour with a little water and add to the mixture. Gradually add the rest of the water, stirring continuously to keep the sauce smooth. Add the Tia Maria and a few drops of vanilla essence. Taste and add honey to sweeten if required. Continue to cook for a few more minutes, stirring all the time.

Put the ice cream into individual dishes and pour the hot sauce on top. Decorate with chopped nuts.

'Chocolate' Mousse

Serves 4

1 teaspoon sunflower
  oil
3 oz (90 g) carob powder
2 tablespoons soft brown
  muscovado sugar
4 tablespoons dry
  Muscadet wine
  (optional)

1 dessertspoon Tia Maria
  (optional)
4 tablespoons water
4 eggs

Put the oil in a saucepan and heat it. Add the sifted
carob powder, sugar, water and wine. If wine and Tia
Maria are not used, add the equivalent amount of extra
water. Stir until the carob and brown sugar dissolve.
Meanwhile, separate the eggs and beat the yolks. Stir
them into the carob mixture, and take it off the heat.
Whip the egg whites very stiffly until they make points.
Fold them into the carob mixture, making sure they are
completely blended. Pour into a serving dish or into 4
individual dishes, and leave to cool.

Small 'Chocolate' Party Cakes

Makes 10 to 12 cakes

3 oz (90 g) plain flour
pinch of salt
1 level teaspoon baking
  powder
1 level tablespoon carob
  powder

2 oz (60 g) butter
1½ oz (45 g) castor sugar
1 egg
a few drops vanilla essence
milk

Sift the flour, salt, baking powder and carob powder
and mix well together. Cream the butter and sugar
together. Whisk the egg and gradually add it to the

175

butter and sugar, beating all the time. Add the flour mixture, vanilla essence and as much milk as is needed for the mixture to be of a soft dropping consistency.

Put this mixture into greased bun tins, leaving room for it to rise. Bake in a moderately hot oven, Gas 5/375° F/190° C, for 15 to 20 minutes.

The cakes can be iced with water icing or butter icing using carob instead of cocoa in both instances.

Butterscotch Creams   *Serves 4*

1 oz (30 g) butter
2 oz (60 g) soft brown
  muscovado sugar
½ pint (300 ml) milk

1 tablespoon cornflour
marshmallows, for
  decoration

Melt the butter and add the sugar and cook until browned. Add the milk and bring to the boil. Blend the cornflour with approximately 1 tablespoon water, add it to the mixture and cook for 1 to 2 minutes, stirring continuously.

Pour into serving dishes or glasses, allow to cool, then decorate with marshmallows.

16

Snacks

Beef and Mushroom Pasties   *Serves 4 to 6*

1 lb (480 g) freshly
  minced beef
1 medium onion, finely
  chopped
2 oz (60 g) oatmeal
4 oz (120 g) mushrooms,
  finely chopped
8 oz (227 g) tin skinned
  tomatoes
1 clove garlic, finely
  chopped

$\frac{1}{4}$ teaspoon mustard paste
$\frac{1}{2}$ teaspoon Worcester
  sauce
pinch of dried mixed herbs
salt and freshly ground
  black pepper
1 lb (480 g) shortcrust
  pastry
1 oz (30 g) butter
milk for glaze

Mix the beef, onion, oatmeal and mushrooms together.
Drain the tomatoes and add them together with the
garlic, mustard, Worcester sauce, herbs and salt and
pepper. Mix everything together well.

Roll out the pastry on a floured board and divide it
into rounds about 5 to 6 in (127 to 153 mm) in diameter.
The pastry should be about $\frac{1}{4}$ in (6 mm) thick. Spoon
the meat mixture on to one half of the pastry rounds.
Dot with butter. Fold the pastry over and nip in the
edges. Brush the tops with milk, prick them and bake
in a hot oven, Gas 7/425° F/220° C, for 10 minutes,

177

then turn down to Gas 4/350° F/180° C. Bake for another 50 minutes.

Alternatively, the meat mixture can be placed in the centre of the pastry rounds. In which case, wet the edges and join them together at the top, making an upstanding frill.

Schlemmerschnitte   *Serves 2*

8 oz (240 g) fillet steak,   2 dessertspoons caviar
  raw   2 small teaspoons chives,
2 slices brown   finely chopped
  buttered toast

Scrape the meat into wafer thin slices discarding all traces of fat. Arrange on the toast and garnish each with a dessertspoon of caviar and a teaspoon of chopped chives.

(Contributed by Jill F. Middleton.)

Steak Tartare   *Serves 2*

6 oz (180 g) minced beef,   dash Tabasco sauce
  raw   salt and freshly ground
1 small onion, finely   black pepper
  chopped   2 eggs
1 dessertspoon French   fresh parsley, chopped
  mustard   2 slices pumpernickel
½ teaspoon paprika pepper   bread, buttered

Mix the beef with the onion, mustard, paprika and Tabasco. Add the salt and pepper. Arrange the mixture

178

into 2 patties, making a well in the centre of each. Break an egg into each well and garnish with chopped parsley. Serve with slices of buttered pumpernickel bread.

Tartar Burger   *Serves 2*

2 hamburger buns
1 clove garlic
6 to 8 oz (180 to 240 g) lean, finely minced beef, raw
1 small onion, finely chopped

2 dessertspoons Worcester sauce
dash Tabasco sauce
salt and freshly ground black pepper
slices of tomato and cucumber, to garnish

Cut buns in half and toast them. Rub the garlic clove over the toasted side of the buns. Mix the minced beef with the chopped onion and Worcester sauce. Season with Tabasco, salt and pepper, then spread the mixture on to the garlicky buns and top with slices of cucumber and tomato.

(Contributed by Jill F. Middleton.)

Cauliflower, Tuna and Cottage Cheese Salad   *Serves 4*

1 green Cox's apple
1 small head of cauliflower
7 oz (198 g) tin tuna fish
4 oz (120 g) carton cottage cheese
1 small clove garlic, finely chopped
1 teaspoon Meaux mustard

1 tablespoon chives, chopped
1 tablespoon cider vinegar
salt and freshly ground black pepper
2 or 3 lettuce leaves or sprigs of watercress, to garnish
slices wholewheat bread

179

Chop the apple into pieces. Break the cauliflower into small florets. Drain the oil from the tuna fish and flake the fish into a bowl. Mix the cottage cheese, finely chopped garlic, mustard, chopped chives and cider vinegar together in a separate bowl. Season with salt and pepper. Fold in the cauliflower florets, tuna fish and chopped apple.

Serve the salad garnished with lettuce or watercress and accompanied by slices of wholewheat bread.

Cottage Delight   *Serves 1 to 2*

4 oz (120 g) cottage
  cheese
1 teaspoon horseradish
  sauce
salt and freshly ground
  black pepper

1 peach
8 white grapes
lettuce leaves
6 black olives

Mash the cottage cheese and stir in the horseradish sauce, season with salt and freshly ground black pepper. Cut the peach into slices, discarding the stone. Halve the grapes and take out the pips. Place 2 lettuce leaves on a plate, arrange the peach slices in a circle and pile the cottage cheese mixture in the middle, topped with the halved grapes and black olives.

Cream Cheese and Caviar   *Serves 4*

4 oz (120 g) cream cheese
1 100 g jar caviar
1 teaspoon dry white wine
2 hard boiled egg yolks

wholewheat toast
slices of cucumber, to
  garnish

180

Mix the cream cheese and caviar together and add the dry white wine. Do not use too much cream cheese or the caviar flavour will be lost. Crumble the hard boiled egg yolks. Cut the wholewheat toast into fingers and pile the caviar and cream cheese mixture on to them. Top with crumbled egg yolks and garnish with twisted slices of cucumber.

Cream Cheese and Date Scones   *Serves 6*

2 oz (60 g) plain flour
3 level teaspoons baking
  powder
pinch of salt
6 oz (180 g) wholewheat
  flour
2 oz (60 g) butter

milk
1 oz (30 g) chopped and
  stoned dates
4 oz (120 g) cream cheese
salt and pepper
butter for spreading

Sift the plain flour, baking powder and salt into a large bowl. Stir in the wholewheat flour. Rub in the butter and add enough milk to make a soft manageable dough.

Knead the dough lightly and roll out on a floured surface to a 6-in (152-mm) round. Divide into scones and place on a greased baking tray. Brush tops with milk and bake at Gas 8/450° F/230° C for about 15 minutes. Cool on a wire tray.

In the meantime, mix the finely chopped dates into the cream cheese and season.

Halve the scones and spread with butter. Fill generously with the date cheese spread. Replace the tops and serve.

Cream Cheese and Chicken   *Serves 4*

4 oz (120 g) cream cheese
salt and freshly ground
  black pepper
dry white vermouth

4 oz (120 g) paper-thin
  slices of cold roast
  chicken

Put the cream cheese in a bowl. Season with salt and pepper. Add as much dry white vermouth as the cheese will take without becoming too thin to spread.

Spread the mixture on to the chicken slices, roll up and secure with a skewer or cocktail stick. Chill in the refrigerator for at least an hour. To serve, cut into bite-size pieces and impale with a cocktail stick.

Mushroom Cheese   *Serves 4*

1 × 15 oz (425 g) can
  consommé soup, jellied
2 level teaspoons gelatine
6 oz (180 g) button
  mushrooms
4 oz (120 g) cream cheese

salt and freshly ground
  black pepper
chopped fresh chives
$\frac{1}{2}$ pint (300 ml) liquid aspic
  jelly

Heat 3 tablespoons of consommé until warm, add the gelatine and continue to heat until dissolved. Set aside a few mushrooms for garnish. Chop the rest very finely and put them in the blender with the jellied consommé, cream cheese and gelatine mixture. Add the salt and pepper and blend until smooth. Pour into dishes and refrigerate until set.

Slice the mushrooms for garnish and arrange them on the mixture together with the chopped chives. Spoon the liquid aspic on top. Chill and serve with brown bread and butter.

Sweet-Sour Chicken Drumsticks   *Serves 4*

4 chicken drumsticks   4 level tablespoons soft
melted butter   brown muscovado sugar
salt and freshly ground   4 to 8 teaspoons thyme
  black pepper   vinegar
4 small onions   paprika

Wipe the drumsticks and brush with melted butter.
Season with salt and pepper. Slice the onions and dip
the slices in the sugar. Cut 4 pieces of cooking foil
large enough to cover each drumstick completely.
Arrange dipped onion slices overlapping on each piece
of foil and sprinkle with the vinegar. Place the chicken
on top. Fold foil up to cover the chicken forming a
small parcel. Bake in a hot oven, Gas 7/425° F/220° C,
for 30 to 45 minutes. Serve chicken with drained onion
on top, sprinkled with paprika pepper.

(Contributed by Jill F. Middleton.)

Chicken Liver Pâté   *Serves 4 to 6*

2 oz (60 g) butter   1 level tablespoon Dijon
2 oz (60 g) onion, finely   mustard
  chopped   sea salt and freshly ground
1 clove garlic, finely   black pepper
  chopped   1 tablespoon dry white
8 oz (240 g) chicken livers   wine (optional)

In a small pan heat the 2 oz (60 g) butter and when
melted add the chopped onion and finely chopped
garlic. Add the livers and cook until they are firm, not

183

allowing the butter to go brown. When cooked, chop the liver mixture, then mash it with the mustard, seasoning and wine to make a rough paste.

Use to fill sandwiches and rolls, or serve on thin brown toast garnished with watercress.

French Chicken Boats

Serves 2 to 4

stale loaf French bread
1 oz (30 g) butter
1 oz (30 g) plain flour
$\frac{1}{4}$ to $\frac{1}{2}$ pint (150 to 300 ml)
   milk
6 oz (180 g) cold chicken,
   chopped

2 oz (60 g) button
   mushrooms, cooked
salt and freshly ground
   pepper
mixed herbs

Cut the loaf in half down the middle and divide into portions. Scoop out the centre of each portion.

Meanwhile, melt the butter in a pan. Remove from the heat, mix in the flour and slowly add the milk. Cook gently, stirring all the time. Add the chopped chicken and mushrooms to the mixture, season with salt and freshly ground pepper and mixed herbs. The mixture should be quite thick.

Fill the bread portions with the chicken mixture, wrap each in foil and cook in a moderate oven, Gas 5/375° F/190° C, for about 20 to 30 minutes.

Anchovy Eggs *Serves 2*

3 eggs
anchovy paste
1 × 1¾ oz (50 g) can
    anchovy fillets
2 slices wholewheat toast

Scramble the eggs in a saucepan in the normal way. In the meantime, toast the bread, and spread it with butter and anchovy paste. Place the scrambled eggs on top of this. Arrange the anchovy fillets on top of the scrambled eggs in a lattice-design and pop the whole lot under a hot grill for a minute or two only, to heat the anchovies. Serve at once.

Crispy Golden Eggs *Serves 2*

5 eggs   finely chopped mixed
salt and pepper   dried herbs
1 cup breadcrumbs   cooking oil
a little plain flour

Hard boil 4 of the eggs. Meanwhile, break the other egg into a bowl and beat it up with a little salt and pepper.

Finely crumble the breadcrumbs, to which you have added a teaspoon of mixed dried herbs.

When the hard boiled eggs are cold, sprinkle them with flour, dip them in the raw egg and then roll them in the breadcrumb mixture.

Fry the eggs quickly in very hot oil and serve with slices of cucumber and sweet pickle.

Curried Eggs   *Serves 2*

1 small onion
2 oz (60 g) butter
¾ pint (450 ml) tomato
  juice
4 eggs

1 dessertspoon curry
  powder
½ teaspoon Worcester
  sauce
2 slices buttered
  wholewheat toast

Finely chop the onion and sauté it in the butter. Put the tomato juice in a separate pan and heat to simmering point. Poach the 4 eggs in the tomato juice. In the meantime add the curry powder and Worcester sauce to the onions and butter and cook quickly, stirring all the time.

When the poached eggs are done, put them on the wholewheat toast and pour the onion-curry sauce over the top. Serve immediately.

Egg Nests   *Serves 1*

4 to 8 oz (120 to 240 g)
  potatoes
knob of butter
2 oz (60 g) cream cheese

salt and freshly ground
  black pepper
½ small onion, finely
  chopped
1 large egg

Peel the potatoes and boil. When cooked, drain and mash with a knob of butter and the cream cheese. Season with salt and pepper and fold in the chopped onion.

Put the mashed potato mixture on a greased ovenproof dish arranged like a nest with a hollow in the middle. Break an egg into the hollow and bake at the top of a pre-heated oven, Gas 6/400° F/200° C, for 20 minutes until the egg white is set.

Piperade *Serves 1*

1 small onion
½ small green pepper
1 skinned tomato
1 oz (30 g) butter

2 eggs
salt and freshly ground
    black pepper

Slice the onion, pepper and skinned tomatoes very thinly. Melt the butter in a saucepan and gently fry the vegetables for a minute or two. Beat the eggs thoroughly and season with salt and pepper. Add them to the mixture, stirring all the time until the eggs begin to set. They should be the consistency of medium scrambled eggs. Serve at once.

Poached Eggs with Spinach *Serves 2*

1 lb (480 g) leaf spinach
salt and freshly ground
    black pepper
2 large eggs
knob butter

Carefully wash the spinach and put into a colander to drain. Put 2 in (5 cm) of water in a large saucepan and bring to the boil, add a little salt and the spinach. Cook quickly for 10 to 15 minutes until tender but not mushy.
    Meanwhile, poach the eggs in an egg poacher or

saucepan of water. Drain the spinach well and serve on to hot plates. Top the spinach with a knob of butter and a poached egg sprinkled with salt and freshly ground black pepper. For a more substantial meal, allow 2 eggs per person.

Scotch Eggs   *Serves 6*

1 × 1¾ oz (50 g) can anchovies
2 tablespoons milk
6 hard boiled eggs
salt and freshly ground black pepper
few drops of Worcester sauce
wholewheat flour
1 beaten egg
1 oz (30 g) toasted brown breadcrumbs
cooking oil for deep frying

Drain the anchovies from their oil and soak them in the milk for 10 minutes. Meanwhile, cut the hard boiled eggs in half and scoop out the yolks.

Take the anchovies out of the milk and mash them up with the egg yolks. Add salt and pepper and a few drops of Worcester sauce. Stuff the mixture into the egg whites and place the 2 halves together again.

Coat the eggs in flour, beaten egg and the fine toasted brown breadcrumbs. Put in the refrigerator for 30 minutes, then deep fry the eggs in very hot fat until golden brown.

Drain and serve.

Tomato Eggs *Serves 2*

1 very small onion
1 dessertspoon cooking oil
1 × 8 oz (227 g) can
　tomatoes
salt and freshly ground
　black pepper

chopped basil
1 dessertspoon tomato paste
few drops Worcester sauce
2 eggs, hard boiled
2 slices fried bread or
　wholewheat toast

Chop the onion very finely and fry in the oil until soft, but do not brown. Separate the tinned tomatoes from the juice and chop them up. Add them to the onions. Season with salt, freshly ground black pepper, basil and tomato paste. Mix together and bring to the boil. Simmer gently, stirring all the time. Add tomato juice as necessary until you have a thick tomato sauce. Add a few drops of Worcester sauce.

Shell the hard boiled eggs, cut in half and put the yolks on one side. Cut the whites in thin strips and add them to the tomato sauce.

Cut the fried bread or wholewheat toast into triangles and arrange around the edges of a plate. Put some of the tomato mixture in the middle, finely chop the yolks of the eggs and add a layer, then another layer of tomato mixture, and so on, ending with a layer of chopped yolk. Serve very hot.

Anchovy Mousse *Serves 4*

8 anchovy fillets
1 teaspoon anchovy paste
6 tablespoons mayonnaise
2 tablespoons single cream
4 standard eggs, hard
　boiled

few drops Tabasco
1 egg white
1 tomato, sliced
watercress

Put the anchovy fillets, paste, mayonnaise and single cream into a blender/liquidizer. Blend to a smooth paste. Peel and chop the eggs finely and add to mixture in liquidizer with a few drops of Tabasco. Blend for a few seconds.

In a separate bowl, whisk the egg white until stiff, then lightly fold the mixture from the blender into it.

Put the mousse into 1 large serving dish or 4 individual dishes and refrigerate for a few hours or until the mixture is firm. Garnish with slices of tomato and watercress, and serve with thin slices of brown toast.

Herring Roes on Toast   *Serves 2*

6 soft roes | 6 fingers of buttered
1½ oz (45 g) butter | wholewheat toast
salt and pepper | freshly chopped parsley

Wash the roes and dry them. Heat the butter in a pan, and fry the roes lightly in it until golden brown. Season with salt and pepper and place on the fingers of buttered toast. Garnish with chopped parsley.

Kipper Quiche   *Serves 4*

8 oz (240 g) kipper fillets | 5 tablespoons cream
½ bunch spring onions | cheese
1 oz (30 g) butter | salt and freshly ground
1 tablespoon plain flour | black pepper
8 fl. oz (240 ml) milk | 1 × 9-in (228-mm) flan
2 eggs | tin lined with uncooked
 | pastry

190

Put the kippers in a bowl of boiling water for about 5 minutes. Meanwhile, wash and trim the spring onions and cut into $\frac{1}{4}$-in (6-mm) lengths.

Put the butter in a saucepan over a low heat. When it has melted, add the spring onions and steam them for 3 to 4 minutes until tender. Drain the kippers and remove any skin.

Put the flour into a blender with the milk, eggs and cream cheese and blend until well mixed and smooth. Flake the kippers and add to the mixture. Add the spring onions and season well with salt and pepper.

Put the mixture into the prepared uncooked pastry case and bake in a moderately hot oven, Gas 6/400° F/200° C, for about 35 minutes.

Kipper Salad *Serves 4*

8 kipper fillets
6 tablespoons French
 dressing (2 parts
 sunflower or olive oil,
 1 part wine vinegar)

salt and freshly ground
 black pepper
1 tablespoon freshly
 chopped parsley

Skin uncooked kipper fillets and lay them in a shallow dish. Pour the French dressing over the fillets and sprinkle with salt and pepper and the chopped parsley. Leave to marinate for about 12 hours or overnight. Serve chilled with wholewheat bread and butter and a green salad.

Salmon Cream   *Serves 4*

1½ oz (45 g) butter
8 oz (240 g) fresh brown
  breadcrumbs
1 × 8 oz (227 g) tin red
  salmon
2 fl. oz (60 ml) single
  cream
1 teaspoon dry white wine

6 oz (180 g) cottage
  cheese
salt and freshly ground
  black pepper
¼ of a cucumber, sliced
2 tomatoes, sliced
2 mushrooms, sliced

Melt butter in frying pan and fry breadcrumbs until browned; place on one side to cool.

Mash the salmon well with the single cream and add the wine. Place two-thirds of the breadcrumbs in a shallow dish. Mash the cottage cheese and spread it on top of the breadcrumbs. Season with salt and pepper. Place the salmon mixture on top and sprinkle the remainder of the breadcrumbs over the salmon. Decorate with the cucumber, tomatoes and mushrooms.

Sardine Pâté   *Serves 6*

1 × 4⅜ oz (124 g) can
  sardines in oil
1 small onion
small bunch chives or tops
  of spring onions
2 oz (60 g) butter
8 oz (240 g) carton
  cottage cheese

4 teaspoons dry white
  wine
1 level teaspoon tomato
  paste
salt and freshly ground
  black pepper
slices of cucumber and
  watercress, to garnish

Chop the sardines, discarding the bigger bones. Chop the onion very finely. Chop the chives or spring onion tops. Cut the butter into small pieces. Put all the chopped ingredients into a blender/liquidizer and add the cheese, wine, tomato paste and salt and pepper. Blend until thoroughly mixed into a smooth paste.

Turn into a bowl and garnish with thin slices of cucumber and pieces of watercress. Refrigerate until needed.

Savoury Kippers   *Serves 2*

2 poached kippers	salt and freshly ground
4 oz (120 g) mushrooms,	black pepper
chopped	bunch of watercress
1 oz (30 g) butter	

Flake the kippers and discard any bones. Sauté the chopped mushrooms in the butter. Add the kipper pieces, season with salt and pepper and cook for a few minutes. Pile on to hot buttered wholewheat toast and serve garnished with watercress.

Savoury Kippers on Toast   *Serves 4*

8 oz (227 g) 'boil in the	*Garnish*
bag' kipper fillets	4 slices cucumber
2 hard boiled eggs	4 stoned olives
little single cream	4 pickled walnuts
salt and freshly ground	fresh parsley
black pepper	
4 slices hot wholewheat	
toast	

Simmer kipper fillets in plastic bag as per instructions. Remove the skin from fish and flake the flesh, mixing in the juice from the bag. Chop the hard boiled eggs and blend them into the mixture with a little cream. Season with salt and pepper. Pile on to slices of hot wholewheat toast and put under the grill for a few minutes to heat through. Garnish with a twist of cucumber and a stoned olive, pickled walnut or a sprig of parsley.

(Contributed by Jill F. Middleton.)

Smoked Haddock Flan   *Serves 4 to 6*

1 small 8 oz (240 g)
  packet frozen pastry
8 oz (240 g) smoked
  haddock fillets
3½ oz (105 g) butter
1 tablespoon capers
1 small onion

4 oz (120 g) cottage
  cheese
1 beaten egg
¼ pint (150 ml) milk
salt and freshly ground
  pepper

Roll out pastry and cook blind in an 8-in (203-mm) pastry case.

Put the haddock in a frying pan, just cover with water, add a knob of butter and poach gently for about 10 to 15 minutes. Drain and break into flakes. Put into flan case together with the capers. Chop the onion very finely and add it to the mixture.

Put the cottage cheese and egg in a bowl, together with the milk and a couple of tablespoons of the fish juices. Beat well together. Season with salt and pepper. Pour into the flan case.

Bake at Gas 5/375° F/190° C for about 40 minutes.

Tuna Fish and Sweetcorn Flan *Serves 4*

Can be made as 1 × 9-in (228-mm) flan or in small individual flan cases.

8 oz (240 g) shortcrust pastry
1½ oz (45 g) butter
1½ oz (45 g) wholewheat flour
½ pint (300 ml) milk
1 × 7 oz (198 g) can sweetcorn, drained
2 standard eggs

1 × 7 oz (198 g) can tuna fish
1 tablespoon tomato paste
½ teaspoon Worcester sauce
salt and freshly ground black pepper
2 tomatoes
a little melted butter

Roll the pastry out into a round about an inch (2.5 cm) wider than the flan tin. Grease the tin, then line it with the pastry, ensuring that it does not crack.

Melt the butter in a pan. Remove from heat and stir in the flour. Gradually add the milk, stirring all the time, over a gentle heat until the sauce is smooth. When the sauce comes to the boil, add the sweetcorn. Beat the eggs up and add them to the sauce and stir the flaked tuna fish into the mixture. Add the tomato paste, Worcester sauce and salt and freshly ground black pepper to taste.

Put the mixture into the prepared flan tin, arrange sliced tomatoes on top and brush the surface with melted butter. Put the flan into a fairly hot oven, Gas 6/400° F/200° C, for the first 10 minutes, then turn the oven down to Gas 4/350° F/180° C and continue baking for another 30 minutes. Cool the flan in the tin.

This flan freezes well.

195

Bumper Decker Sandwiches   *Serves 6*

2 eggs, hard boiled
2 tablespoons thick
  mayonnaise
12 slices wholewheat
  bread
4 oz (120 g) butter
4 oz (120 g) tuna fish,
  mashed

3 oz (90 g) cucumber,
  finely sliced
4 oz (120 g) carton
  cottage cheese
salt and pepper
3 oz (90 g) tinned red
  peppers
parsley

Chop the hard boiled eggs and mix into a paste with the mayonnaise (this can be done in a blender).

Spread the thickly sliced bread with butter. Place 3 slices butter side up on a flat surface. Spread each slice with mashed tuna fish, topped with slices of cucumber, and season lightly. Top each slice with another slice of buttered bread (butter side up). Spread with seasoned cottage cheese, and the red pepper slices. Top this with another 3 slices of bread, butter side up, spread with the hard boiled egg mayonnaise mixture and seasoning. Finish with 3 more slices of bread, this time butter side down. Press lightly, wrap each in foil and refrigerate for about 45 minutes. Cut each decker into 2 triangles. Serve garnished with parsley.

Cream Cheese Sandwiches   *Serves 2 to 4*

4 oz (120 g) cream cheese
1 teaspoon grated
  horseradish
$\frac{1}{2}$ teaspoon Worcester
  sauce
salt and freshly ground
  black pepper

1 dessertspoon single
  cream
1 dessertspoon chopped
  fresh parsley
wholewheat bread

Put the cream cheese in a bowl, beat in the horseradish, Worcester sauce and salt and freshly ground black pepper. Add enough cream to make a good spreading consistency. Add the chopped parsley. Sandwich between thin slices of wholewheat bread. This is also good on wholemeal biscuits and crackers.

Cream Cheese and Walnut Sandwiches   *Serves 2 to 4*

cayenne pepper
4 oz (120 g) carton cream
  cheese
3 oz (90 g) walnuts, finely
  chopped or
  rough-ground

brown bread and butter
watercress

Mix the cayenne pepper into the cream cheese to taste. Add the walnuts. Mix thoroughly and spread the mixture on slices of brown bread and butter and make into sandwiches. Garnish with watercress.

French Sardine Sandwich   *Serves 2*

small loaf French bread
1 × 4⅜ oz (124 g) can
  sardines in oil
mayonnaise

Cut the French bread into 2 pieces approx. 6 in (153 mm) long and split them lengthways. Toast the bread on one side only (not the cut side). Now put the toasted bread, cut side up, in the grill pan without

197

the wire rack. Place the sardines on the bread and spoon over all the sardine oil so that the bread is nicely saturated. Grill for 3 to 5 minutes. Remove and spread with thick mayonnaise. Serve immediately.

N.B. If you are very hungry you may use 2 cans of sardines!

(Contributed by Jill F. Middleton.)

Walnut Cheese Open Sandwich   *Serves 2*

slices of pumpernickel
   bread
2 pickled walnuts
4 oz (120 g) cream cheese
few drops Worcester sauce

freshly ground black
   pepper
1 fl. oz (30 ml) single
   cream
chopped parsley

Lightly butter the pumpernickel bread. Mash the pickled walnuts and blend them with the cream cheese. Add a few drops of Worcester sauce, the freshly ground black pepper and enough cream to make a smooth, spreadable mixture. Spread on to the slices of pumpernickel and garnish with chopped parsley.

Cream of Cauliflower and Almond Soup   *Serves 4 to 6*

1 cauliflower
1¾ pints (1 l) milk
1 chicken stock cube
1 oz (30 g) ground
   almonds

salt and freshly ground
   black pepper
1 oz (30 g) toasted
   almonds, flaked
3 fl. oz (90 ml) cream

198

Wash the cauliflower and break into florets. Cook in ¾ pint (450 ml) of the milk to which the stock cube has been added. Cook quickly for about 10 minutes. Liquidize the mixture and return it to the saucepan; add the ground almonds and the rest of the milk until the soup is the consistency you want. Stir all the time. Season with salt and freshly ground black pepper.

Garnish with the flaked toasted almonds and serve with a spoonful of cream poured into the centre of each bowl.

Cream of Mushroom Soup　　　　　　　　　*Serves 4*

8 oz (240 g) mushrooms	1½ pints (900 ml) milk
1 small onion	salt and freshly ground
1 small clove garlic	black pepper
2 to 3 oz (60 to 90 g)	2 fl. oz (60 ml) cream
butter	4 teaspoons freshly
1 oz (30 g) plain flour	chopped parsley

Wash the mushrooms (there is no need to peel them), and chop them very finely. Also finely chop the onion and the garlic. Put the butter in a saucepan and when it has melted, add the onion and garlic. Cook them gently until the onion is transparent. Do not brown. Add a quarter of the mushrooms, put a lid on the saucepan and cook gently for a few minutes. Stir in the flour and gradually add the milk, stirring all the time. When half the milk has been added, put in the rest of the mushrooms. Cook for 5 minutes and then add the rest of the milk.

Cook gently for another 15 to 20 minutes, stirring regularly. Season with salt and pepper.

Serve with a spoonful of cream floating on the top of each bowl of soup, garnished with the chopped parsley and some roughly ground black pepper.

Cream of Watercress Soup   *Serves 4 to 6*

2 small onions
2 bunches watercress
1½ oz (45 g) butter
1 oz (30 g) flour
2 pints (1.2 l) milk

1 chicken stock cube
salt and freshly ground
   black pepper
4 to 6 teaspoons fresh
   cream

Chop the onions very finely. Put half a bunch of watercress on one side. Chop the other 1½ bunches. Melt the butter in a saucepan and fry the chopped onions and watercress until the onions are translucent. Add the flour and mix into a paste. Gradually add the milk, stirring all the time. Crumble in the stock cube. Bring the soup to the boil and simmer for about 10 minutes. Season with salt and pepper. Now sieve or liquidize the soup and return it to the saucepan.

Chop the remaining ½ bunch of watercress roughly and add it to the soup just before serving. Add a teaspoon of fresh cream to each helping.

Spinach Layer Pancakes   *Serves 4*

2½ lb (1.2 kg) fresh
  spinach
1½ oz (45 g) butter
1½ oz (45 g) plain flour
8 fl. oz (240 ml) milk
1 large egg
salt and freshly ground
  black pepper

garlic
4 oz (120 g) cottage
  cheese
2 oz (60 g) cream cheese
2 oz (60 g) sour cream
chopped chives

Make 6 thin pancakes. Wash the spinach and cook quickly for 5 to 6 minutes. Drain thoroughly and put on one side. Do not chop.

To make the sauce, melt the butter in a saucepan and stir in the flour; add the milk, stirring all the time until the sauce is smooth and comes to the boil. This sauce will have a very thick consistency. Beat the egg well, then whisk it into the sauce. Season the mixture with salt and freshly ground black pepper.

Finely chop the clove of garlic. Add it to the cottage cheese and cream cheese. Put the mixture in the blender and blend to a smooth paste. Add salt and pepper. Stir the cheese mixture into the sauce. The whole will be very thick indeed now. Take a deep ovenproof dish and grease it with a little butter. Put a pancake at the bottom of the buttered dish, place some spinach on it and spread a layer of the cheese mixture on top of this, then another pancake and so on until the dish is filled up. Finish with a pancake spread with the cheese mixture, pour the sour cream over the lot and sprinkle with the chopped chives or spring onions.

Bake in a moderate oven, Gas 5/375° F/190° C, for 45 to 50 minutes.

Cut the pancakes into wedges in the dish before lifting out each helping.

17

Beverages

Non-Alcoholic

Apple and Cucumber shake   *Serves 2*

2 sweet apples
$\frac{1}{3}$ of a cucumber
2 tablespoons cider
    vinegar
$\frac{3}{4}$ pint (450 ml) cold water

Peel and core the apples. Cut into pieces and put in the
blender. Cut a few slices of cucumber and put on one
side. Peel the rest and add to the blender together with
the cider vinegar and water. Blend until smooth. Add
more water if necessary. Serve chilled in tall glasses.
Decorate with a slice of cucumber from those put on
one side.

Apple Ginger Fizz

unsweetened apple juice
ground ginger
soda water
slices of unpeeled apple

Fill each glass half full of unsweetened apple juice. Sprinkle on ground ginger to taste. Fill rest of glass with soda water. Stir well and decorate with a slice of unpeeled apple.

Brose   *Serves 4*

1 lb (480 g) apple cores
1 pint (600 ml) water
1 teaspoon oatmeal
1 teaspoon clear honey

Put the apple cores, including pips, into the water. Add the oatmeal and honey and boil the whole mixture up. Let it stand until cool, then strain and serve.

'Chocolate' Egg Nog   *Serves 2*

1 dessertspoon clear honey
$\frac{3}{4}$ pint (450 ml) milk
3 teaspoons carob powder
1 beaten egg

Dissolve the honey in a little of the milk, then whisk or blend together all the ingredients. Serve chilled.

'Chocolate' Milk Shake (1)   *Serves 2 to 4*

2 dessertspoons clear
   honey
1 pint (600 ml) milk
1½ oz (45 g) carob powder

Melt the honey in a little hot water, then combine it with the milk. Pour in the carob powder and whisk well. Alternatively, put the whole lot in a liquidizer. Serve chilled in tall glasses.

'Chocolate' Milk Shake (2)   *Serves 1*

½ pint (300 ml) milk   1 dessertspoon carob
small teaspoon clear honey   powder
                            ¼ teaspoon vanilla essence

Put all ingredients in a liquidizer or blender and blend until smooth. Serve hot or cold.

'Chocolate' Milk Shake (3)   *Serves 2*

1 dessertspoon carob   1 pint (600 ml) milk
   powder   2 small teaspoons clear
1 fl. oz (30 ml) sunflower   honey
   oil   a few drops vanilla essence

Dissolve the carob powder in the oil and add a little milk. Put over a gentle heat for a few minutes to cook the carob. Take the mixture off the heat and blend it with the rest of the milk, honey and the vanilla essence. This can be served hot or cold.

Coffee Nog *Serves 1*

½ pint (300 ml) milk   a few drops of coffee
1 egg yolk   essence
½ teaspoon honey

Mix together well in a blender. Any flavouring of your
choice can be substituted instead of the coffee.

Elderberry Drink

fresh elderberries
water
a few cloves
clear honey

Wash the elderberries and pick the berries off the
stems. Use equal amounts of berries and water and blend
in the liquidizer until smooth. Sweeten to taste
with honey and add a few whole cloves. Put in a large
jug with lots of ice.

Hot Mulled Apple Juice *Serves 4 to 6*

2 pints (1.2 l)
   unsweetened apple juice
1 × 2½-in (63-mm) piece
   cinnamon stick
5 whole cloves

Put the juice, cinnamon and cloves in a saucepan and
bring to the boil. Reduce the heat and simmer the
mixture for about 20 minutes. Strain and serve hot in
mugs.

Hot Mulled Pineapple Juice   *Serves 4 to 6*

2 pints (1.2 l)   3 or 4 cloves
  unsweetened pineapple   pinch of ground nutmeg
  juice   pinch of ground allspice
1 × 2-in (50-mm) piece
  cinnamon stick

Pour the juice into a saucepan and add the cinnamon
stick, cloves and spices. Heat until boiling, then reduce
the heat, put a lid on the saucepan and simmer the
mixture for about 20 minutes. Remove from the heat,
take out the cinnamon stick and cloves and serve hot in
mugs.

Hot Vegetable Juice   *Serves 1 to 2*

1 × 12½ fl. oz (355 ml)   salt and freshly ground
  can vegetable juice   black pepper
1 clove garlic

Empty vegetable juice into a saucepan and add the
clove of garlic sliced into 3 or 4 pieces. Bring to the boil
and simmer for a few minutes. Add salt and pepper to
taste. Serve hot.

Iced Tea   *Serves 4 to 6*

Earl Grey tea   slice of lemon (optional)
ice cubes or crushed ice   or sprigs of fresh mint
                                and slices of cucumber

Make a pot of tea, using Earl Grey tea (2 small teaspoons per person). Let it stand for a few minutes then pour it through a strainer into a glass full of ice cubes or crushed ice. For those who can take it, serve with a slice of lemon; for those who can't, put a sprig of fresh mint and a slice of cucumber into the glass before serving.

For a stronger iced tea, use fresh tea to make the ice cubes.

This is a very refreshing drink.

Melon Refresher   *Serves 2 to 4*

1 small cantaloupe melon	crushed ice
unsweetened pineapple juice	sprigs of fresh mint

Peel the melon and discard the seeds. Cut into pieces and liquidize with a little of the unsweetened pineapple juice. Put into a large jug with plenty of crushed ice. Thin down the mixture with unsweetened pineapple juice and garnish with sprigs of fresh mint.

Minty Apple Cup   *Serves 4*

1 pint (600 ml) unsweetened apple juice	ice cubes
$\frac{1}{2}$ pint (300 ml) mint tea	sprigs fresh mint
	slices of cucumber

Mix well together. Add lots of ice cubes, sprigs of fresh mint and slices of cucumber. If you can eat citrus fruits, this is delicious with slices of fresh lemon.

Night-Time 'Chocolate' *Serves 1*

1 to 2 teaspoons carob
  powder
¼ pint (150 ml) milk

2 tablespoons water
a few drops of vanilla
  essence

Put the carob powder in a cup and mix it with the water until a smooth paste is obtained. Meanwhile, put the milk in a saucepan to heat up. Just before the milk boils, take it off the heat and pour it on to the carob paste, stirring all the time. Return the complete mixture to the pan for a few minutes and add a few drops of vanilla essence.

Pineapple Brose *Serves 2*

2 glasses unsweetened
  pineapple juice
2 Cox's or Granny Smith
  apples

clear honey to taste
cocktail cherries

Put the pineapple juice in the liquidizer. Peel and core the apples, chop them and add them to the liquidizer. Blend until smooth. Add the honey. Blend again. Serve chilled in tall glasses decorated with cocktail cherries.

Pineapple Cocktail *Serves 4*

½ bunch fresh watercress
1 × 19 fl. oz (540 ml) can
  pineapple juice
ice cubes

Cut off most of the stems and add the fresh watercress leaves to a large can of pineapple juice. Put into a blender and liquidize until smooth. This makes a lovely combination of sweet and bitter. Serve with ice.

Summer Sparkler

pineapple juice
ginger ale
ice cubes made from
   frozen pineapple juice

glacé cherries
slices of cucumber

For each person, fill a tumbler or beaker with one-third pineapple juice and two-thirds ginger ale. Add pineapple ice cubes, glacé cherries and slices of cucumber.

(Contributed by Jill F. Middleton.)

Sunshine Shake   *Serves 2*

4 fl. oz (120 ml) canned
   pineapple juice
$\frac{1}{2}$ pint (300 ml) ice-cold
   milk

fresh mint
pineapple cubes

Mix the pineapple juice and ice-cold milk together and shake or whisk until the mixture froths. Pretty up with a sprig of mint and a few cubes of pineapple.

(Contributed by Jill F. Middleton.)

Tiger's Milk   *Serves 2 to 4*

1 pint (600 ml) milk
1 tablespoon brewer's
    yeast
$\frac{1}{2}$ × 19 fl. oz (540 ml) can
    pineapple juice
1 dessertspoon molasses

Mix well together in a blender and serve chilled.

Alcoholic

Adonis   *Serves 1*

1 fl. oz (30 ml) Italian dry
    vermouth
2 fl. oz (60 ml) lime
    cordial
2 drops Angostura bitters

Stir briefly over ice cubes.

Apple Julep   *Serves 4*

1 pint (600 ml)
    unsweetened apple juice
$\frac{1}{2}$ pint (300 ml)
    unsweetened pineapple
    juice

$\frac{1}{4}$ pint (150 ml) dry white
    wine
$\frac{1}{4}$ pint (150 ml) soda water
fresh mint

Mix all the ingredients together. Pour into a large container with plenty of ice and decorate with sprigs of fresh mint.

Champagne Fruit Punch *Serves 4 to 6*

1 fresh pineapple   honey syrup
1 quart (1.2 l) Chablis or   1 bottle champagne
  dry white wine

Peel the pineapple and cut into cubes. Marinate in 1 quart (1.2 l) Chablis or dry white wine for 12 hours in an ice box or freezer. Add simple honey syrup (melted honey) to taste, plus 1 bottle champagne. Serve chilled.

Champagne Julep *Serves 1*

1 sprig fresh mint
slices of cucumber
champagne
1 lump sugar

Put mint and cucumber into a wineglass with ice and pour champagne over, stirring all the while, then add the sugar.

Everyman's Bubbly

white wine, chilled
soda water

Simply mix one-third wine to two-thirds soda water. Chill well. If you like it sweet, try Graves or Sauterne, if you prefer it dry, try Hock or Chablis.

(Contributed by Jill F. Middleton.)

Ginger Grape Cocktail   *Serves 3 to 4*

½ pint (300 ml) dry white wine
½ pint (300 ml) dry white grape juice
½ pint (300 ml) soda water
1 teaspoon powdered ginger
slices of cucumber

Mix well together and serve with ice and slices of cucumber.

Martini Tonic   *Serves 1*

dry Martini bianco
tonic water
slice of cucumber
ice cubes

Mix dry Martini with tonic water, add a slice of cucumber and lots of ice.

Moonlight Fizz   *Serves 2 to 4*

white of 1 egg
1 wineglass gin
1 teaspoon castor sugar
20 drops Angostura bitters
crushed ice
soda water

Beat up white of egg well. Mix gin, sugar, Angostura bitters and crushed ice. Add the egg white and shake well. Strain into cocktail glasses and fill up with soda water.

Rhine Wine Cobbler   *Serves 2*

1½ tablespoons sugar
½ wineglass of soda water
1½ wineglass Rhine wine

Mix and serve chilled.

Shandy Gaff

light ale
American dry ginger or
    ginger ale
crushed ice

Equal parts light ale and American dry ginger or ginger ale. Mix together well, add crushed ice and serve.

Sherry Cobbler (if tolerated)   *Serves 4*

½ pint (300 ml) dry sherry   1 bottle soda water
1 oz (30 g) castor sugar   ice
sprig of mint   slices cucumber

Mix sherry and sugar together and add a few leaves of fresh mint. Add the soda water, crushed ice and slices of cucumber.

White Wine Punch   *Serves 8*

1 bottle dry white   two large cups strong tea
  vermouth $\frac{1}{3}$ pint (200 ml) sugar syrup
1 bottle dry white wine   1 syphon soda water

Mix and refrigerate. Decorate with slices of cucumber, and serve chilled.

White Wine Cup   *Serves 4*

1 bottle white burgundy or   powdered sugar, to taste
  any dry white wine   thin slices of fresh
1 wineglass dry white   pineapple
  vermouth   fresh sprigs of mint
1 bottle club soda   lots of ice

Mix wine, vermouth and club soda together. Sweeten with the sugar and serve with lots of ice, decorated with the slices of fresh pineapple and sprigs of mint.

Appendix

I: THE MIGRAINE TRUST

THE MIGRAINE TRUST was founded in 1965 to raise funds on a national basis for migraine research and to act as the authoritative medical body in that field. It is located at 45 Great Ormond Street, London WC1 (Tel: 01 278 2676).

The Medical Advisory Council of the Trust is composed of distinguished specialists in the various branches of medicine concerned with migraine, whose expert knowledge is applied to the planning of research projects.

The Trust opened its first City Migraine Clinic in 1970 to provide emergency and consultative facilities for migraine sufferers and to allow clinical observation of cases in acute attack. Between 1970 and 1973 this Clinic alone treated over 6000 patients. It was replaced in 1973 by the Princess Margaret Migraine Clinic at 22 Charterhouse Square, London EC1, which is run in association with St Bartholomew's Hospital.

Any person suffering a severe attack of migraine can go to this Clinic for immediate help. It is open from 9.45 a.m. to 4 p.m. during weekdays

Other hospitals which have a special interest in

migraine are the following:

The Charing Cross Hospital, Fulham Palace Road, London W6

The National Hospital, Queen Square, London WC1

King's College Hospital, Denmark Hill, London SE5

The Birmingham Eye Hospital, Birmingham

Neurological Unit, Northern General Hospital, Ferry Road, Edinburgh 5

Southern General Hospital, Glasgow

The Royal Surrey County Hospital, Guildford, Surrey

Hull Royal Infirmary, Anlaby Road, Hull

The Radcliffe Infirmary, Oxford

II: ATTACK FORMS

Name .... Date ....

                                Day of week ....

                                Time of onset ....

                                Duration ....

Day of cycle ....   Days before next menstruation .....

During the 24 hours BEFORE the attack:
(1) Did you have any special worry, overwork or shock?
(2) What had you done during the day?
     Normal work?   Unusual activity?   Extra tired?
(3). What food had you eaten and when?

Breakfast ....   Time ....

....

Mid-morning ....   Time ....

....

Lunch ....   Time ....

....

Mid-afternoon ....   Time ....

....

Supper ....   Time ....

....

Evening ....   Time ....

....

Bedtime ....   Time ....

....

What do you think caused this attack?

218

II: ATTACK FORMS

Name .... · Date ....

Day of week ....

Time of onset ....

Duration ....

Day of cycle .... Days before next menstruation .....

During the 24 hours BEFORE the attack:
(1) Did you have any special worry, overwork or shock?
(2) What had you done during the day?
    Normal work? Unusual activity? Extra tired?
(3). What food had you eaten and when?

Breakfast .... Time ....

....

Mid-morning .... Time ....

....

Lunch .... Time ....

....

Mid-afternoon .... Time ....

....

Supper .... Time ....

....

Evening .... Time ....

....

Bedtime .... Time ....

....

What do you think caused this attack?

219

II: ATTACK FORMS

Name .... Date ....

Day of week ....

Time of onset ....

Duration ....

Day of cycle .... Days before next menstruation .....

During the 24 hours BEFORE the attack:
(1) Did you have any special worry, overwork or shock?
(2) What had you done during the day?
    Normal work? Unusual activity? Extra tired?
(3). What food had you eaten and when?

Breakfast .... Time ....

....

Mid-morning .... Time ....

....

Lunch .... Time ....

....

Mid-afternoon .... Time ....

....

Supper .... Time ....

....

Evening .... Time ....

....

Bedtime .... Time ....

....

What do you think caused this attack?

II: ATTACK FORMS

Name .... Date ....

Day of week ....

Time of onset ....

Duration ....

Day of cycle .... Days before next menstruation .....

During the 24 hours BEFORE the attack:
(1) Did you have any special worry, overwork or shock?
(2) What had you done during the day?
    Normal work? Unusual activity? Extra tired?
(3). What food had you eaten and when?

Breakfast .... Time ....

....

Mid-morning .... Time ....

....

Lunch .... Time ....

....

Mid-afternoon .... Time ....

....

Supper .... Time ....

....

Evening .... Time ....

....

Bedtime .... Time ....

....

What do you think caused this attack?

II: ATTACK FORMS

Name . . . . Date . . . .

Day of week . . . .

Time of onset . . . .

Duration . . . .

Day of cycle . . . .   Days before next menstruation . . . . .

During the 24 hours BEFORE the attack:
(1) Did you have any special worry, overwork or shock?
(2) What had you done during the day?
    Normal work? Unusual activity? Extra tired?
(3). What food had you eaten and when?

Breakfast . . . .   Time . . . .

. . . .

Mid-morning . . . .   Time . . . .

. . . .

Lunch . . . .   Time . . . .

. . . .

Mid-afternoon . . . .   Time . . . .

. . . .

Supper . . . .   Time . . . .

. . . .

Evening . . . .   Time . . . .

. . . .

Bedtime . . . .   Time . . . .

. . . .

What do you think caused this attack?

II: ATTACK FORMS

Name .... Date ....

Day of week ....

Time of onset ....

Duration ....

Day of cycle .... Days before next menstruation .....

During the 24 hours BEFORE the attack:
(1) Did you have any special worry, overwork or shock?
(2) What had you done during the day?
    Normal work? Unusual activity? Extra tired?
(3). What food had you eaten and when?

Breakfast .... Time ....

....

Mid-morning .... Time ....

....

Lunch .... Time ....

....

Mid-afternoon .... Time ....

....

Supper .... Time ....

....

Evening .... Time ....

....

Bedtime .... Time ....

....

What do you think caused this attack?

III: FREQUENCY CHARTS

	Jan.	Feb.	Mar.	Apr.	May	June
1						
2						
3						
4						
5						
6						
7						
8						
9						
10						
11						
12						
13						
14						
15						
16						
17						
18						
19						
20						
21						
22						
23						
24						
25						
26						
27						
28						
29						
30						
31						
Total						

July	Aug.	Sept.	Oct.	Nov.	Dec.

Name:

Year:

III: FREQUENCY CHARTS

	Jan.	Feb.	Mar.	Apr.	May	June
1						
2						
3						
4						
5						
6						
7						
8						
9						
10						
11						
12						
13						
14						
15						
16						
17						
18						
19						
20						
21						
22						
23						
24						
25						
26						
27						
28						
29						
30						
31						
Total						

July	Aug.	Sept.	Oct.	Nov.	Dec.

Name: _____

Year: _____

Bibliography

Abrahamson, E. M., M. D., & Pezet, A. W., *Body, Mind and Sugar*, Holt, Rinehart & Winston, New York 1951

'Amines & Migraine', *British Medical Journal*, **693**, 23 December 1967

Arch, *Biochemistry*, **85**, 487, 1959

Blau, J. N., & Cumings, J. N., 'Method of Precipitating & Preventing Some Migraine Attacks', *British Medical Journal*, **2**, 1242, 1966

Cochrane, Professor A. L., CBE, MA, MB, FRCP, Editor, *Background to Migraine – Third Migraine Symposium 24–25 April, 1969*, Wm Heinemann Medical Books Ltd, London 1970

Cugh, C. S., University of California, 'Measurement of Histamine in Californian Wines', *Journal Agricultural Food Chemistry*, **19**, 241–244, 1971

Cumings, J. N., Editor, *Background to Migraine*, Wm Heinemann Medical Books Ltd, London 1973

Dalessio, D. J., MD, 'Dietary Migraine', *American Family Physician*, **6:60**, 5 December 1972

Dalton, Dr K., 'Do-it-Yourself', *Migraine News Letter*, British Migraine Association, London, April 1975

Dalton, Dr K., *The Menstrual Cycle*, Penguin Books, Harmondsworth, Middlesex 1969

Dalton, Dr K., 'Migraine in General Practice', *Journal Royal College of General Practitioners*, **23**, 97, 1973

228

Dalton, Dr K., 'Migraine – A Personal View', *Proceedings of the Royal Society of Medicine*, **66**, 263, London, March 1973

Dalton, Dr K., *The Pre-Menstrual Syndrome*, Wm Heinemann Medical Books Ltd, London 1964

Dalton Dr K., 'Progesterone Suppositories & Pessaries in Treatment of Menstrual Migraine', *Headache*, **12**, 4, 151, 1973

Davis, Adelle, *Let's Eat Right to Keep Fit*, George Allen & Unwin, London 1961

Davis, Adelle, *Let's Get Well*, Unwin Books, London 1974

Davis, Francyne, *The Low Blood Sugar Cookbook*, Bantam Books Inc., New York and Corgi, London 1974

Epstein, M. T., Hockaday, J. M., & Hockaday, T. D. R., Radcliffe Infirmary, Oxford, 'Migraine and Reproductive Hormones Throughout the Menstrual Cycle', *The Lancet*, 8 March 1975

Gerras, Charles, Editor, *Natural Cooking – The Prevention Way*, Rodale Press, Emmaus, USA 1972

Hanington, Edda, M. D., *Migraine*, Priory Press Ltd, London 1973

Hanington, Edda, M.D., 'Preliminary Report on Tyramine Headache, *British Medical Journal,* **2**, 550–551, 1967

Hockaday, J. M., Williamson, D. H., & Alberti, K. G. H. M., 'Effects of Intravenous Glucose on Some Blood Metabolites and Hormones in Migrainous Subjects', *Background to Migraine*, Cumings, J. N., Editor, Wm Heinemann Medical Books Ltd, London 1973

Journal American Medical Association, **188**, 1108, 1964

Journal of Institute of Brewers, 1958: 257; 1971: **77**, 446–450; 1972: **15**, 25–29; 1972: **78**, 322–326

Kent, Howard, 'Yoga Techniques – The Treatment of Migraine and High Tension Headache', A Report on a

Controlled Programme with Migraine Sufferers', Yoga for Health Clubs, London 1975

Kinderlehrer, Jane, *The Art of Cooking with Love and Wheatgerm*, Rodale Press, Emmaus, USA 1977

Kohler, Marianne, *The Secrets of Relaxation*, Souvenir Press, London 1972

Luce, Gay Gaer, *Body Time*, Maurice Temple Smith, London 1972

Mackarness, Dr R., *Not All in the Mind*, Pan Books Ltd, London 1976

Marquardt, P., & Werringloer, H. W., 'Toxicity of Wines Food Cosmet', *Toxicol*, **3**, 803–810, 1965

Migraine, Office of Health Economics, London 1972

Migraine and Diet, Nutritional Services Quarterly Review, National Dairy Council, London, January 1975

Migraine News, Journal of the Migraine Trust, 1975

Moffet, A. M., Swash, M., & Scott, D. F., 'Effect of Chocolate in Migraine, A Double-Blind Study', *Journal of Neurology, Neuro-Surgery and Psychiatry*, **37**, 445–448, 1974

Moffet, A. M., Swash, M., & Scott, D. F., 'Effect of Tyramine in Migraine, a Double-Blind Study, *Journal of Neurology, Neuro-Surgery and Psychiatry,* **35**, 496, 1972

New York Times Natural Foods Cookbook, Souvenir Press Ltd, London 1972

Pearce, J., Ron, M. A., & de Silva, K. L., 'Further Studies of Carbohydrate Metabolism in Migraine', *Background to Migraine*, Cumings, J. N., Editor, Wm Heinemann Medical Books Ltd, London 1973

Prevention Magazine, Rodale Press, London and Emmaus, USA

Sander, M., Youdin, M. B. H., & Hanington, E., 'A Phenylethylamine Oxidising Defect in Migraine', *Nature*, **250**, 335, 1974.

Steincrohn, Peter J., M.D., *Low Blood Sugar*, Allison & Busby, London 1973

Somerville, B. W., 'The Role of Progesterone in Menstrual Migraine', *Neurology, Minneapolis,* **21**, 853, 1971

Wheaton and Stewart, *Analytical Biochemistry,* **12**, 585, 1965

Index

232

234